W0113744

"An admirable achievement. This is an innovative book of many parts with a rich diversity of voices, each one skillfully articulating how IFS can work its wonders in consultation and supervision. Open-hearted collaboration is key to the practice of IFS, and the authors are often vividly transparent in their writing, bringing the multi-faceted consultative work alive on the page. I believe all supervisors and consultants, whether IFS-trained or not, will benefit from a study of this pioneering text."

Jim Holloway, *independent counselor and supervisor (BACP senior accredited)*

"Through a wealth of wide-ranging case studies, the book's contributors demonstrate how bringing unconscious processes into awareness can bring clarity and resolve impasses. Particularly striking is the supervisory stance of respectful curiosity and use of their own internal system as a guide to the work. Although aimed at IFS practitioners, there is much in this very readable book that will speak to practitioners from other approaches."

Els van Ooijen, *author of* Clinical Supervision Made Easy

"*Internal Family Systems Therapy: Supervision and Consultation* is a truly important contribution to the IFS literature as well as to the entire supervisory endeavor. The breadth and scope of the chapters is matched by the depth of the material presented. The open-hearted and non-shaming approach of IFS supervision will help any clinician provide a safe and enlightening experience for their supervisees."

Lisa Spiegel, MA, LMHC, *author of* Internal Family Systems Therapy with Children

"For those committed to getting the model inside, this is a crucial addition to the IFS library. *Internal Family Systems Therapy: Supervision and Consultation* has many chapters in which authors model tracking their own parts and discerning what information from parts to share in the consultation process. This modeling helps consultees do the same, bringing authentic communication skillfully into the consultation room and then into the delivery to clients in therapy, education, and coaching. Chapters on implicit bias, training, and consultation to non-dominant groups give needed depth to the reader's use of the model. Each author gives clear digestible steps toward enhanced practice."

Rina Dubin, *IFS lead trainer*

"*Internal Family Systems Therapy: Supervision and Consultation* is a primer to effective supervision using the IFS model. It's also a guide to looking at therapeutic stuckness through the lens of the client's parts, the clinician's parts, the relational dynamics, as well as the supervisor's parts. Case examples of supervision with particular populations, including those with eating disorders, BIPOC, veterans, and more make this usable, applicable, and understandable. This book is a must read for clinicians who want to do supervision in the IFS model."

Marla Silverman, PhD, *certified IFS therapist, psychologist, and faculty at The Gestalt Center*

"A fascinating read, even for readers (like myself) who find themselves curious about IFS and with great respect for IFS-trained colleagues, but who haven't undertaken a formal IFS training. This is a timely and refreshing read and a valuable collection of not just the theory but the application of theory *in practice*. It offers rich glimpses and a multitude of voices exploring many facets of IFS supervision and consultation from racism and serious illness, to working with military veterans, and an opening interview with IFS founder Richard C. Schwartz. Much respect to all the contributors for a rich and engaging read."

Emma Palmer, *counselor, body psychotherapist, supervisor, author, www. kamalamani.co.uk*

"Full of technical guidance about IFS consultation and supervision, this practical volume is highly accessible for beginners and experienced IFS therapists alike. Drawing links and distinctions between the provision of IFS therapy and IFS supervision/consultation, the authors subtly but profoundly shift the emphasis from those *receiving* IFS to those *providing* it. With an emphasis on humility and Self-energy, the author of each chapter touches on a vital aspect of the IFS model providing the reader with an abundance of real-world examples, principles, and strategies neatly presented in the context of a range of sound theoretical models."

Shaun Dempsey, PhD, *clinical psychologist in private practice, certified IFS therapist and approved clinical consultant*

"IFS consultants and trainers continually invite students and consultees to explore their internal systems to gain clarity, courage, and, most importantly, access to inner wisdom and Self-energy. Each chapter in *Internal Family Systems Therapy: Supervision and Consultation* offers robust case material and outlines the IFS perspective on countertransference. Even though our goal as IFS therapists and practitioners is Self-leadership, each case comes with its own unique challenges. How we approach issues related to the therapist's parts may change depending on a wide variety of circumstances. Whether new to IFS, already an IFS supervisor or working in other models, this book offers creative ideas and support for therapists as they navigate complexity while supporting clients to heal."

Toni Herbine-Blank, *IFS senior trainer and co-author of* Internal Family Systems Couple Therapy Skills Manual

"As the global need for IFS professionals continues to grow, so does the need for Self-led, competent, and inclusive IFS consultants and supervisors.

Informed by decades of collective experience, this diverse collection offers clinical, theoretical, and personal applications and a depth of wisdom that cannot be understated. This invaluable resource helps IFS consultants clarify and develop their supervisory framework while respectfully challenging personal biases and assumptions. This book will strengthen and expand the next generation of Self-led IFS healers and deserves to be required reading for all IFS consultants and supervisors. I am delighted to recommend and welcome this important contribution to our IFS family."

Laura Schmidt, LMFT, *certified IFS therapist and consultant for certification, AAMFT-approved supervisor*

Internal Family Systems Therapy

Internal Family Systems Therapy: Supervision and Consultation showcases the skills of Richard C. Schwartz and other leading IFS consultants and supervisors. Using unique case material, models, and diagrams, each contributor illustrates IFS techniques that assist clinicians in unblending and accessing Self-energy and Self-leadership. The book features examples of clinical work with issues such as bias, faith, sexuality, and sexual hurts. Individual chapters focus on therapist groups, such as Black Therapists Rock, and on work with specific populations, including children and their caregivers, veterans, eating disordered clients, therapists with serious illnesses, and couples. This thought-provoking book offers an opportunity for readers to reflect on their own supervision and consultation (both the giving and receiving of it). It explores what is possible and preferable at different stages of development when using the IFS model.

Emma E. Redfern is a certified IFS therapist and approved IFS clinical consultant. She specializes in supervising those who are transitioning to becoming IFS therapists and offers workshops on IFS supervision.

Internal Family Systems Therapy

Supervision and Consultation

Edited by
Emma E. Redfern

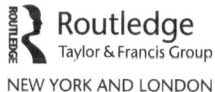
Routledge
Taylor & Francis Group

NEW YORK AND LONDON

Cover image: © Kathy Nettles Art, Devon, UK

First published 2023
by Routledge
605 Third Avenue, New York, NY 10158

and by Routledge
4 Park Square, Milton Park, Abingdon, Oxon OX14 4RN

Routledge is an imprint of the Taylor & Francis Group, an informa business

Library of Congress Cataloging-in-Publication Data
Names: Redfern, Emma E., editor.
Title: Internal family systems therapy : supervision and consultation / edited by Emma E. Redfern.
Description: New York, NY : Routledge, 2023. |
Includes bibliographical references and index. |
Identifiers: LCCN 2022004854 (print) | LCCN 2022004855 (ebook) | ISBN 9780367482640 (paperback) | ISBN 9780367482657 (hardback) | ISBN 9781003044864 (ebook)
Subjects: LCSH: Psychotherapy patients--Family relationships. | Systemic therapy (Family therapy) | Family psychotherapy.
Classification: LCC RC489.F33 I585 2023 (print) | LCC RC489.F33 (ebook) | DDC 616.89/14--dc23/eng/20220218
LC record available at https://lccn.loc.gov/2022004854
LC ebook record available at https://lccn.loc.gov/2022004855

ISBN: 978-0-367-48265-7 (hbk)
ISBN: 978-0-367-48264-0 (pbk)
ISBN: 978-1-003-04486-4 (ebk)

DOI: 10.4324/9781003044864

Typeset in Bembo
by Taylor & Francis Books

Dedicated to Moira Jean (Ma), with whom I shared a love of words, books, and reading.

Contents

Illustrations

Figures

Tables

Contributors

Fran Booth, LICSW, is an IFS trainer and a certified IFS therapist and consultant. A clinician for more than 40 years, she integrates multiple modalities into her IFS framework, especially psychodynamic, attachment theory, and body-focused ways of working. As a speaker and seminar leader, Fran has conducted over 100 workshops across the globe. She graduated from Cornell University with honors and from Simmons School for Social Work.

Jeanne Catanzaro, PhD, is a clinical psychologist who has worked with eating disorders and trauma over the past 20 plus years. She has written two chapters on using IFS to treat eating disorders, one in *Innovations and Elaborations in Internal Family Systems Therapy* (2017) and another in *Trauma-Informed Approaches to Eating Disorders* (2019). More recently her focus has expanded beyond eating disorders to help clients explore more generally the cultural and personal legacy burdens that affect all of our relationships with food and our bodies.

Sharon Cooper, PhD, is a clinical psychologist and IFS-trained therapist who has worked with veterans and their families since 2002 and has been using the IFS model of therapy since 2011. Along with her colleague, Dr. Kimberly Corey, she has presented at annual IFS conferences on using IFS with military veterans and their families. As part of her responsibilities, she provides IFS-informed supervision to psychology trainees and, since 2018, provides IFS-informed consultation to licensed mental health clinicians who work exclusively with veterans and their families.

Kimberly Corey, PhD, is a clinical psychologist who has worked with veterans and their families for nearly two decades. With her colleague, Dr. Sharon Cooper, she has presented on this subject multiple times at the annual IFS Conference. In her clinical practice, Dr. Corey works with veterans of all generations (from WWII to the recent conflicts in Iraq and Afghanistan) and provides training and supervision to VA psychology interns and post-doctoral fellows. In addition, Dr. Corey provides both formal and informal consultation to colleagues interested in how IFS-informed techniques can build rapport, improve clinical outcomes, and reduce clinician burnout.

Ann E. Drouilhet, LICSW, LMFT, is a founding partner of Family Development Associates of Framingham, MA, where she has practiced couples and family therapy for over 30 years. For the last 12 years her work with couples and as a consultant to other therapists has been dedicated to the application of the IFIO model (Intimacy From the Inside Out), developed by Toni Herbine-Blank. She is a co-lead trainer for the IFIO training program and maintains her certification as an approved supervisor for the AAMFT, which she first earned in 1998.

Tamala Floyd, MSW, LCSW, is a certified IFS therapist and trainer, trauma specialist, life coach, consultant, and speaker with over 25 years of experience. She consults with Black Therapists Rock to bring IFS to the BIPOC population. She grew up in Marina del Rey and Los Angeles, CA. Her work focuses on women's trauma and relationship issues. She provides individual coaching to women, business consultation to therapists, and speaks on subjects related to challenges in mother and adult child relationships and the effects of emotional wounds on mothering. She contributed a chapter to the book *Fiercely Speaking* (2019), edited by Audra Lowray Upchurch.

Pamela K. Krause, LCSW, is a senior lead trainer for the IFS Institute who leads all three levels of IFS training. She and Toni Herbine-Blank developed the online training program the IFS Online Circle. She presents on the use of IFS with children and adolescents nationally and internationally and delivered an IFS Continuity Program addressing the use of IFS with this population. She has written three published chapters, one in *Internal Family Systems Therapy: New Dimensions* (2013), and co-authored two, one in *EMDR Therapy and Adjunct Approaches with Children* (2013) and one in *Innovations and Elaborations in Internal Family Systems Therapy* (2017).

Kate Lingren, LICSW, has been in practice for nearly 40 years. She has studied and taught IFS for the past 14 years and is a lead trainer for IFIO (Intimacy From the Inside Out), the application of IFS in couple therapy, developed by Toni Herbine-Blank. She is on the faculty of Boston College School of Social Work, where she teaches a graduate course on IFS. Kate is co-founder, with Percy Ballard, of Bigotry From the Outside In (BFOI), a model that uses IFS to access, understand, and bring healing to parts that hold biased beliefs. She is committed to working toward a more just and inclusive world.

Liz Martins, MSc, is a certified IFS therapist and approved clinical consultant. She was appointed as a co-lead trainer in 2021 following extensive international experience as a PA/lead PA. Liz has a private practice near Bath, UK. During the global pandemic beginning in 2020, she and Emma Redfern began offering online introductory trainings for those wanting to integrate IFS into their supervision practices. Although IFS is her primary modality, she is also a certified Sensorimotor Psychotherapist and EMDR practitioner. With colleagues, Liz organizes the annual IFS Open Space for the IFS community in the UK and beyond.

Roberta Rachel Omin, LCSW, has been in private practice since 1985 and is a certified IFS and IFIO therapist and consultant with a specialty in treating individuals, couples, and families with chronic, acute, or life-threatening illnesses. She has presented on this topic at national IFS conferences and local IFS gatherings in Boston, New York, Ann Arbor, the Gestalt Center of Long Island, and the Clinical Social Work Society. Roberta's published articles include "To Reveal or Not to Reveal: When the Therapist has a Serious Illness" (*Psychotherapy Networker*, 2020) and "When the Therapist Becomes the Medical Patient" (*Journal of Social Work in End-of-Life & Palliative Care*, 2014).

Emma E. Redfern, MA, MBACP (Snr Accredited), is a certified IFS therapist and approved IFS clinical consultant. She specializes in supervising those who are transitioning to becoming IFS therapists. During the global pandemic beginning in 2020, she and Liz Martins began offering online introductory trainings for those wanting to integrate IFS into their supervision practices. A number of her articles have been published, including the peer-reviewed "The Drama Triangle and Healthy Triangle in Supervision" (*The Irish Journal of Counselling and Psychotherapy*, 2021). Emma's online practice is based in Devon, UK.

Dan Reed, PhD, LPC, became a counselor educator in 2018 after teaching physics for ten years. In the spring of 2019, Dan received his PhD in counselor education and supervision. His interest in how IFS informs ongoing development for psychotherapists and psychotherapist educators led to his doctoral thesis, *Internal Family Systems Informed Supervision: A Grounded Theory Inquiry*. Currently, Dan is an assistant trainer for the IFS institute (IFS-I), an IFS-I approved clinical consultant, and a certified IFS therapist. He operates a private practice in San Antonio, TX, offering support for leaders, consultation for IFS therapists and IFS consultants, and counseling.

Richard C. Schwartz, PhD, began his career as a systemic family therapist and an academic at the University of Illinois and at Northwestern University. He is now on the Faculty of the Department of Psychiatry at Harvard Medical School, and he is a Senior Fellow of the Meadows treatment center in Arizona. Grounded in systems thinking, Dr. Schwartz developed the Internal Family Systems model (IFS) in response to clients' descriptions of various parts within themselves. A featured speaker for national and international professional organizations, Dr. Schwartz has published many books and over 50 articles about IFS.

Robin Shohet is a British pioneer in the field of supervision. He has been supervising and training supervisors since 1976 and has published widely, including co-authoring *In Love with Supervision* (2020) and four editions of *Supervision in the Helping Professions* (1st ed., 1989). His edited works include *Passionate Supervision* (2008) and *Supervision as Transformation* (2012).

Mary Steege is a certified Internal Family Systems therapist, licensed marriage and family therapist, and pastor in the Presbyterian Church, USA. She is drawn to the Internal Family Systems model for the way in which it facilitates spiritual healing and recovery, as well as life-giving connection with the Divine. A frequent presenter on IFS and the Christian tradition, she is also co-author, along with Richard C. Schwartz, of *The Spirit-led Life: A Christian Encounter with Internal Family Systems* (2010).

Martha Sweezy, PhD, is a part-time assistant professor at Harvard Medical School and a program consultant and supervisor at the Cambridge Health Alliance. She has co-authored numerous books on IFS, including *Internal Family Systems Therapy* (2nd ed., 2020); *Internal Family Systems Therapy: New Dimensions* (2013); *Internal Family Systems Skills Training Manual: Trauma-Informed Treatment for Anxiety, Depression, PTSD & Substance Abuse* (2017); and *Internal Family Systems: Couple Therapy Skills Manual* (2021). She has also published peer-reviewed articles on IFS, including for the *Journal of Psychotherapy Integration* and the *American Journal of Psychotherapy*. She maintains a therapy and consultation practice in Northampton, MA.

Nancy Wonder, PhD, is a licensed psychologist in private practice in Tallahassee, FL, with over 15 years of experience with Internal Family Systems. She has served as a co-lead trainer for the IFS Institute and is currently a senior faculty member for Intimacy From the Inside Out. Dr. Wonder offers consultation to therapists learning IFS and IFIO. She has worked with sexual abuse treatment her entire career and has had a chapter published in *Internal Family Systems Therapy: New Dimensions* (2013), entitled "Treating Pornography Addiction with IFS." She has presented the IFS Continuity Program module IFS Treatment for Sexual Abuse: Victims and Perpetrators.

Ray Wooten, PhD, LPC-S, is a professor at Texas A&M University in San Antonio, TX. Ray has over 30 years of experience as a counsellor educator and clinical supervisor. He is a registered somatic educator and movement therapist focusing on soul-centered practices, facilitating self-awareness and conscious embodiment. He has presented nationally and internationally on topics ranging from Self-led supervision to embodied approaches to social justice.

Foreword

As someone who has been supervising since the 1970s and training and writing on the subject with my wife and partner Joan, we are often asked by authors to provide written contributions to their books. I am pleased to do so for this book for several reasons. First, it had such an immediate and interesting impact on me in that it made me want to know more about IFS. Second, reading Emma Redfern's book I noticed I was able to self-supervise, a tribute to the clarity in the chapters and within the methodology itself. Added to that, I found myself naturally integrating some of the techniques and approaches in the book when supervising. We are invited to look at our cases with a different eye, and the idea of protectors, exiles, and the Self makes intuitive sense (see the Glossary). Finally, I share with IFS and this edited book's authors the view that the best resource you have as a supervisor is to know yourself and help the therapist to know themselves. As a supervisor, I hold the idea that "there is no client," a radical idea that says we only have the therapist's view of the client, which is bound to be affected by countertransference or, in IFS language, the therapist's parts.

For Joan and me, supervising is a valid endeavor to be enjoyed, and this book showcases many dedicated professionals doing what they love doing. IFS professionals (both supervisors and supervisees) and non-IFS professionals will find much within these pages to enjoy and by which to be challenged. The book makes an important contribution to the IFS library and to the field of supervision generally.

Robin Shohet, August 2021

Preface

Editorial Choices

Terms

This book includes both sets of terms for the processes that therapists engage in when they discuss their clinical work with a trusted professional, whether supervision, supervisor, supervisee or consultation, consultant, consultee. The authors had carte blanche to use the terms that apply to their practice and to explain them in their chapters, or not. Yes, this may be irritating and confusing for some readers—I get that. Parts are entitled to their responses. And I hope it won't get in the way of you engaging with the pearls of wisdom and gems of experience contained in what follows. I have many pragmatic and practical parts, and we chose to not make this a book of debate about terms. Similarly, I have parts that value IFS highly because it truly honors difference. The co-existence of differentiated parts in the presence of Self is a thing of beauty, and I wasn't about to dictate that I wanted all authors to use the same terms for their varied endeavors. I chose early on to welcome the varied voices, emphases, and contexts of the authors.

However, I have decided to enforce across the whole book certain choices: when referring to a person's racial identity, the book uses "Black" and "White" rather than "black" and "white"; when reference is made to a person's gender, the term "cisgender" may be used to indicate the writer's gender identity corresponds with the sex the person had or was identified as having at birth; and US-English spelling (e.g., –ize rather than –ise), punctuation, and phrasing ("How do you feel toward?" rather than "How do you feel towards?") are used throughout.

Various styles are used to indicate parts' inner communications and beliefs depending on the contexts in which they are shared.

In Chapter 2, Dan Reed and Ray Wooten have chosen to highlight the mutually reciprocal nature of the Self-*and*-part relationship as distinct from the more conventional IFS construct of "Self-to-part" relationship. "Self-and-part" is indicated through the use of a dash that is slightly longer than a hyphen (an "en" dash): Self–part.

A list of abbreviations is included in the preliminary pages, and there is a Glossary at the back of the book that explains some of the key terms and core concepts for those less familiar with Internal Family Systems therapy.

Difference

Accepting and appreciating difference is an important value for me. For this reason, I have not homogenized the chapters as much as some readers would expect, have become used to, or would prefer. This is because, as with the practice of IFS therapy, we all come to supervise in our own way or ways (some of us have a wider range of practice than others) and with our own favourite phrases, preferences, and so on. I did not want to edit away individual differences. To me this richness and diversity of relationship and offering are important; each of us needs and wants different things and responds differently at different times in our professional career or journey. The ability to make healthy choices is a sign of Self-leadership, or, as Cece Sykes is known to say, "Choice could well be the 9th C of Self-leadership" (Cece Sykes, personal communication, August 18, 2021).

Diversity

Although a pleasing variety of voices is represented within the following pages, there are voices missing. Psychotherapy demographics continue to be dominated by Western, White, educated, middle-to-upper class, cisgendered females with Western, White, educated, middle-to-upper class, cisgendered males dominating leadership roles and by way of being founders, figureheads, and established authors. Currently, IFS demographics narrow things even further by being dominated by and from the USA (although I know the IFS Institute is actively working to bring about change). This book reflects that wider bias. It offers both a blessing and a lost opportunity. It is a blessing because the wisdom and length and depth of experience of Richard Schwartz, Pamela Krause, and other lead trainers are being brought to the wider and developing IFS communities. Also, having such people on board meant that a longstanding publisher of repute took a risk on me, an unknown author, and on what is a potentially risky publication, in terms of sales.

I feel the lost opportunity, however, in the lack of authorship by those who are less represented in the psychotherapy and IFS communities, perhaps particularly in leadership roles, which include supervisory or consultatory and training positions. Therapists and consultants from the BIPOC community, those who identify as LGBTQIA, and those residing outside the USA are under-represented. I am immensely grateful to Tamala Floyd, Kate Lingren, and my UK colleague, Liz Martins, for trusting me and themselves enough to write their chapters, thus filling some of that void or absence of important voices. It is my hope that we can each take this book into our communities within the larger community in order to inspire and encourage others to contribute in ways that are meaningful to them and to those they serve.

So, sadly, some readers will not find themselves fully represented, neither in the authors of the chapters nor by the supervisees who feature in the chapters. This is a source of regret for me because my own healing and growing journey was given momentum by finding aspects of myself represented in psychotherapy texts. It is my hope that you might find some aspects of yourself reflected in the struggles, successes, and transformations within the following pages.

Lastly, please note that, whether noted or not in each chapter, all case material is disguised, fictionalised, adapted, or conflated into a composite, and if reproduced or reconstructed from reality, then written permission for its use in this book was sought and given. If you believe you and your material are represented here without your permission, I suggest that this may be a testament to the skills of the writers and the universality of the issues and themes illustrated.

Attribution

When using in-text citation and references, I have done my best to attribute material to the appropriate sources. However, when one is immersed in IFS, as I and the authors have been for some time through different media (reading, teaching, writing, watching webinars, listening to recordings, attending conferences, having and offering supervision and consultation, etc.), it is not always easy to acknowledge and reference the original source. Much of what we know is "in the ether." If I have erroneously attributed anyone's material or failed to provide an important citation, I apologize and assure any injured parties that it was not intentional. Attempts will be made to rectify such errors (and others) in future editions.

Caveat Emptor, or Buyer Beware

It goes without saying that this book is not intended as a substitute for supervision (consultation, mentoring, or grandparenting, etc.) with an experienced and qualified professional. Nor is it a substitute for training in IFS and in supervision.

Although I have sought to highlight—and some authors have risked showing—the common humanity and fallibility of supervision professionals, much of the case material shows best-case examples. Please consider wisely how you use what you read (inside your own system and in the outside world). Some of your parts may feel encouraged, others self-flagellating, still others judgmental and critical of what they read. Some parts may want to risk something new with their supervisors or with their supervisees. Please go gently. If you try something new, please use your reflective skills and curiosity to assess what works, what doesn't, or what might suit your developmental needs and those with whom you work.

Lastly, some of the contributors are more experienced in IFS and in supervision than others. I chose this mix on purpose, partly to inspire, motivate, and inform those who may think that only lead IFS trainers can do this work. As of the time of writing, that is not the case. Nor is there a one-size fits all model of IFS supervision. In some senses there is—and has been—a creative void in this area, which I and others are responding to in our different ways. Some of what we have created may stand the test of time, some may not, and much may be revised. As a psychotherapy professional or an IFS professional working outside of a psychotherapy context, it is incumbent upon you to use the material as well and as wisely as you can in line with your experience, training, competence, and ethical framework as well as within your own contexts and relationships. My hope is that this book will serve existing and future supervisors. I thank you in advance for your consideration, and should you wish to drop me a line, you may do so via my website: www.emmaredfern.co.uk.

Emma E. Redfern

Acknowledgments

I start by acknowledging the founder of IFS, Richard C. Schwartz. Without the dedication and abilities of his parts as well as his persistence, perspective and Self-led vision for IFS to reach the world, this book would not exist. I am so grateful to have spent time as his student and now as a collaborator by interviewing him for inclusion in this book. Next, I wish to thank Martha Sweezy and Ellen L. Ziskind for their patience, creativity, and skill in producing the two books that inspired this one: *Internal Family Systems Therapy: New Dimensions* (2013) and *Innovations and Elaborations in Internal Family Systems Therapy* (2017). On a more personal note, I wish to thank Ellen for joining with me in commissioning most of the contributors to this book. Rina Dubin also played a significant role in bringing potential authors to our attention, and I extend our joint thanks to her. I thank each of the contributors for their dedication to this project and for sharing their time, energy, and of themselves with me and the reader. I am grateful also to those who wanted to contribute to the book but for whom it was not possible for whatever reason. Others in the IFS community to whom my personal thanks are extended include Sarah Stewart, Paul Ginter, Sue Richmond, Lisa Spiegel, Gayle Williamson, Paula Biles, Rosa Chilari Barb Cargill, and Mike Elkin. I was PA (program assistant) for the first time with Barb and am forever moved at her bringing to my awareness that I might have something to offer the wider IFS community.

Closer to home, I would like to thank the IFS UK community, past and present. These include Ginny Bennett, who with Nicola Hollings first brought Richard Schwartz to these shores; Irene Davies, who brought IFS to Broxbourne, near London, just as I found the confidence and desire to PA; and Nicola Hollings and Olivia Lester, who are at the helm of IFS UK supported by Sue Smith, Liz Calvert, and Krissy Tingle. Thanks also to all those I had the pleasure of meeting, working with, and getting to know whether as a student, Program Assistant, supervisor, workshop leader, or at IFS Open Space. Special appreciation goes to Liz Martins, IFS colleague and collaborator, with whom I have been offering introductory trainings on integrating IFS into supervision.

Thanks also to Debra Hayden and Andrew Forrester for their long-term, non-IFS, and valuable supervisory support. Appreciation also to my supervision trainers at the Centre for Supervision and Team Development, Bath and London: Judy Ryde, Robin Shohet, and Joan Shohet (previously Wilmot). I owe much to my many therapists and therapy trainers over the years and hope you know who you are and how much I value what we have been through together.

On a more personal note, I wish to thank my husband, Martin Redfern, especially for generously sharing his IT and editing skills; friends in Devon, UK, for contributing in different ways to the buoyancy and energy needed to complete this project: Kathy Nettles, the Greenes, the Brights, the Wednesday Club, Sue Hunter, Tracey Wills, and Andrew Broadhead. Special thanks also to the team of talented professionals who help keep my old bones on the road: Caroline Whyman (Qigong), Helen Watts (Myofascial Release), Alexandra Williams (Osteopathy), and Jo Hamilton (TRE). My thanks also to other friends and colleagues who, along the way, gave support and validated my aspirations to get published: Graeme Smith, Wendy Pope, Linda Winn, Peter Lane, Luke Gray, Emma Palmer, and John Nettles.

Finally, I extend gratitude to Anna Moore, Grace McDonnell, Ellie Duncan, and Priya Sharma at Routledge; Emma Steele of Emphasis Creative, Devon, UK, who designed all the figures, which add that something extra alongside the written word; and Kathy Nettles (www.kathynettlesart.com) for use of the original artwork, which created a meaningful and attractive cover.

Abbreviations

AAMFT	American Association for Marriage and Family Therapy
ACEs	Adverse Childhood Experiences
ACT	Acceptance and Commitment Therapy
BACP	British Association for Counselling and Psychotherapy
BFOI	Bigotry From the Outside In
BIPOC	Black and Indigenous People of Color
BTR	Black Therapists Rock
CBT	Cognitive Behavioral Therapy
DBT	Dialectical Behavioral Therapy
DID	Dissociative Identity Disorder
EMDR	Eye Movement Desensitization and Reprocessing
IFIO	Intimacy From the Inside Out, the application of IFS to couple therapy
IFS	Internal Family Systems
IFS-I	Internal Family Systems Institute
LCSW	Licensed Clinical Social Worker
LGBTQIA	Lesbian, Gay, Bisexual, Transgender, Queer and/or Questioning, Intersex, and Asexual and/or Ally
LGBTQI+	an umbrella term for all those who have non-normative gender identity or sexual orientation
LICSW	Licensed Independent Clinical Social Worker
LMFT	Licensed Marriage and Family Therapist
LPC	Licensed Professional Counselor
LPC-S	Licensed Professional Counselor with Training Supervision
MBACP	Member of the British Association for Counselling and Psychotherapy
MBCT	Mindfulness-Based Cognitive Therapy
PA	Program Assistant (on IFS-I trainings)
pH	'Psychotherapeutic H'
PTSD	Post-Traumatic Stress Disorder
TA	Transactional Analysis
TSRC	Traumatic Stress Research Consortium, Kinsey Institute
VA	Veterans Health Administration

Introduction

Martha Sweezy

In Internal Family Systems (IFS), therapy for me is therapy for you too. As you help me welcome my Self, who will soothe my protectors and heal my exiles, you do the same for your protectors and exiles. If you are my therapist and one of your protectors reacts to one of my parts, you have the opportunity to find your exile and heal it. If you are my supervisee, we both have the opportunity – with the help of many clients in absentia since we therapists are always drawing on what we learn from clients – to notice our protectors and find our exiles. If you supervise a group of therapists, everyone has the opportunity to notice their protectors and find their exiles – with the help of many clients in absentia – when one participant speaks. This is true because systems (the psyche, dyads, groups) nest and mirror each other, which means the IFS treatment process can be applied to systems at all levels. As the authors of this book emphasize and illustrate with case examples, IFS therapy and supervision are multisystem inquiries.

Emma E. Redfern, this volume's editor, interviews Richard C. Schwartz on his philosophy of supervision. His approach includes helping therapists to view clients as tor-mentors, who are skilled at detecting the therapist's parts, and to apologize if the therapist's parts intrude on therapy. He talks about the importance of not fearing clients' extreme parts, not being afraid of getting it wrong ("Just ask."), and knowing how to defuse suicide parts (which he describes). Although Schwartz will cover technique when supervising, he declares himself a minimalist whose overarching goal is to empower therapists to trust their Self.

Dan Reed and Ray Wooten offer a detailed overview of consultation from an IFS perspective. They suggest contracting at the outset of each consultation session and recontracting as the session goes along. They describe a number of technical options for consulting, including engaging in role-plays, listening to recordings together, the therapist giving a case presentation, discussing skills or offering observations, tracking Self-leadership, and guiding the therapist in a U-turn. Reed and Wooten also detail methods for unblending, which appear as an Appendix at the back of the book.

Liz Martins, who collaborates and teaches about IFS supervision with Emma Redfern, writes about a framework they developed, which they call

DOI: 10.4324/9781003044864-1

"The Fs and Ps of IFS Supervision," a systemic approach that can be scaled up to organizational, cultural, and global contexts or scaled down to an individual's internal system. Their Fs and Ps include having a systemic frame, partnering with the model, being patient with stuckness, staying present through Self-energy, accessing fluency with persistence, and being creatively playful.

Pamela K. Krause describes and illustrates her three-pronged consultation method with therapists who see children and their parents. In addition to listening as the therapist explores what their parts feel toward the client, she gives the client representation in the consulting process by listening as if she is the client and/or their parents and shares that perspective with the therapist. Thus, when Krause consults, she gives every stakeholder – the client's parts, the client's caregiver's parts, the therapist's parts, and the consultant's parts – a voice.

Ann E. Drouilhet describes the consultation process for the IFS approach to couple therapy, called Intimacy From the Inside Out (IFIO), starting with contracting and orienting the therapist to practices like presenting a case, formulating a clinical question, and doing a role-play. She points out that facilitating the U-turn is as crucial in consultation as it is in therapy, explains the nature of certain common polarizations between couples and in couple therapy, and suggests (since therapists can be blind to their own missteps and blended parts) that video recordings can be an invaluable tool for consultation.

Tamala Floyd explains and illustrates her various supervisory and programing hats, including consulting on IFS to the organization Black Therapists Rock, for whom she developed and runs a five-session consultation group to prepare program assistants and participants for IFS Level 1 trainings. She explains how she adapted the IFS model for BIPOC therapists and their BIPOC and LGBTQIA clients with an eye to their long history of oppression and trauma in the United States. In addition, she explains why legacy burdens are especially important for the BIPOC population.

Jeanne Catanzaro illustrates a Self-led approach in consulting to therapists who are working with clients who have eating disorders or disordered eating, an arena that is rife with power struggles, inside and out. She points out that all therapists work with eating issues in some way, not least because we have our own concerns and burdens related to the body, health, and eating. She includes examples of therapists getting satisfaction when their parts or their clients' parts transform.

Nancy Wonder examines the challenges facing therapists and consultants who work in the arenas of sexual abuse, sexual offending, and sexual compulsivity. These include inadequate education in graduate schools, the cultural influence of the Puritan and Catholic roots of Western culture, the booming business of online pornography, and the pervasive presence of sexualized advertising. She suggests that unblending will help therapists and consultants alike bring their personal beliefs and feelings about sexuality to consciousness with the aim of being more Self-led.

Kate Lingren writes about implicit and explicit bias, microaggressions, and shame, illustrating how to address bias both internally, in the consultant, and with therapists in consultation. Since the question is *when* not *if* bias will arise in any one of the people involved (consultant, therapist, or client) regarding any number of issues, she highlights the importance of contracting to include the topic at the outset of a consultation relationship.

Mary Steege reviews some typical challenges for therapists who work with religious or spiritual clients, including rigid managers who feel tasked with saving the soul and the firefighter parts who threaten their project. She highlights some external constraints that may affect a client's ability to engage in therapy and frustrate the therapist. And she points out that the concept of the Self is compatible with many religious and spiritual practices, making it a very accessible way for this population to resolve inner conflict.

Sharon Cooper and Kimberly Corey explain how the military culture of the United States, the realities of war, and the importance of mission over personal safety can be obstacles for returning veterans in their transition back to civilian life. Typical challenges include feeling confused, guilty, and angry about war experiences and feeling fearful that others will not be able to understand. The authors point out that therapists who work with this population may have parts who feel inadequate, helpless, and challenged by the job of listening to combat veterans recount the traumas they witnessed and experienced. They prioritize helping therapists access their Self.

Roberta Rachel Omin speaks to the topic of the therapist who is ill or dying. She relates her own "crisis of authenticity" when she became ill as well as her explorations in this often-overlooked area of a therapist's personal and professional life. She conducted in-depth interviews with over 100 therapists and clients. Based on that information, in addition to her own experience, she developed and describes some "Principles of Contextual Self-Led Disclosure." Her aim is to help therapists traverse the terrain of illness and impending death from the heart, seeking to do the least harm and honoring the opportunity for reparative attachment in the therapeutic relationship.

Fran Booth spells out the kind of contractual agreements a therapist can make with a consultant, either including personal exploration or just help-ing parts unblend and identifying trailheads. She illustrates how an IFS consultant can help a therapist who has contracted for personal exploration to follow the trailhead of their own reactivity with certain kinds of clients to find their protectors and help their exile unburden.

Emma E. Redfern introduces a map or model of IFS supervision devel-oped with Liz Martins called "The 8 Facets of IFS Supervision." These are the Self, the client's system, the therapist's system, the supervisor's system, the flow of the IFS model, the therapeutic relationship, the supervisory relationship, and the wider systems. The author includes questions for supervisor and supervisee self-reflection in each category, offers some diagrams in addition to clinical examples, and shares some personal as well as professional experience.

In IFS, all roads lead to exiles. But along the way specific populations have unique challenges, therapists and consultants have parts, and pitfalls abound. When we educate ourselves about challenges, we empower our anxious or judgmental parts to relax, separate, and trust the Self. These chapters illustrate common themes for IFS supervision along with diversity and creativity in application. We humans are always different and always similar. Our parts feel and think differently from each other and from other people, but the psyche functions in the same way across the board. As a result, between the experience-near methods of inquiry in IFS and the all-inclusive bird's eye view of the Self, we can, like a good novelist, get to some broad truths. IFS supervision is an invaluable part of that endeavor.

1 An Interview with Richard C. Schwartz

Richard C. Schwartz and Emma E. Redfern

Introductions

Introducing The Book

REDFERN: *Let me tell you about my vision for the project. I'm hoping this will be a book that gives examples of what actually happens in IFS supervision in different contexts and with different client groups. Each chapter is going to be by a different IFS consultant or pair, and they are going to write something about their supervision or consultation practice with their client group or in their context. What I'm hoping for here is to talk about what you do in your consultation. You share that on the IFS Continuity Program, but not everybody who reads this book is going to be aware of the Continuity Program, so they won't necessarily see you doing that. Does that sound reasonable?*
SCHWARTZ: Yeah, sounds good.

Getting an Introduction to the Client and the Work

I notice that when you first meet with the supervisee on the Continuity Program, you ask them to share some of the "backstory." Can you say more about that?

I like to listen to get something about the client's context and symptoms and then to get the history of what they've been doing with IFS and in terms of where they are stuck. So that much, yes.

Yes, and I guess one of the things I find difficult sometimes when I'm supervising is if somebody is used to working in a particular way, they sometimes give a lot of content, so it is about achieving a balance—not too much but enough.

Yeah. You know, because I find that most stuck points are because of the therapist's parts, I don't need as much content about the client. So, if someone is going on and on, at some point I'll stop them and I'll say some version of, "Tell me what this client brings up in you," and we try and get past the stuck point.

DOI: 10.4324/9781003044864-1

Box 1.1

IFS Continuity Program: an online membership program providing monthly teaching videos and live webinars over a four-month, content-specific module. Open to those who are enrolled in or have completed IFS Level 1 training and those who have already participated in the IFS Online Circle.

Validating the Therapist's Work

Yes, great. Also, I've noticed, as an example from when you were working with a couple of supervisees this week on the IFS Continuity Program (Schwartz, 2020), that you also do things like share from your experience.

Okay, yes, one person was working with a ritual abuse survivor and both therapists were working with clients that it's really difficult to work with. So, in a situation like that, primarily, I'll try to recognize that.

Yes, you will verbally recognize that with them, validate them.

Exactly, not only recognize that the work is difficult but, secondly, focus on the lengths to which the therapist has gone out of their way to really help the client, and how great that is, and how this is a marathon. It's not a sprint with clients like that … because a lot of people, you know they get stuck and then they start to criticise themselves for being stuck, and so I'm trying to counter those critics in the beginning, and you know therapists are scared to come to me a lot of the time, because I'm the master and admitting that they are having trouble using the model is challenging sometimes.

So, in the beginning I'm just trying to reassure all those therapist parts that they are doing fine and that I used to get stuck in very similar places. I know these kinds of clients, and it's really important to let them be your teachers.

Working with Stuckness

Therapist Parts Getting in the Way

So, sometimes in supervision you might work with the parts that come up in the therapist.

Yes, I'd say 80 percent of the time my supervision goes there. Maybe not quite that much, maybe 70 percent of the time. Because I find that as therapists access Self and unburden the parts that are being triggered by these situations, they know what to do next. I don't have to tell them things. They just get a lot of clarity about what had been stuck. Sometimes they'll come to me and say, "I know that I need to do this thing, but I can't get through it," and then the part that we need to work with is clear. But then other times they don't know, and they blame it on the client. Then after we've done some work, they can see, "Oh it really isn't about the client," and that it's about their countertransference to the client.

Sometimes you might work with protectors in the therapist and sometimes you might even do a piece of work with their exiles if their protectors allow?

Yes, many times, you wind up negotiating for permission to go to an exile and heal it, and then the protectors all relax and now they're not so extreme about the client.

Having our Clients be Our Tor-mentors

That makes me think more about what the goals of consultation might be, and one of the goals might be helping therapists to access more of their own Self-energy?

Yes, my philosophy in all the years of being a therapist and consultant, and what I try to convey to trainees is, "Use your clients, let them be your tor-mentors—with a hyphen between the *tor* and the *mentor.*" The assumption is that there are clients—not all clients, but some clients—who are incredibly good teachers. They trigger us the most, and typically they have qualities that are somehow related to people that we were betrayed by or maybe trusted in the past or something. This happened in my own experience—I'm a very different person because I allowed my clients to teach me that way. When I would get triggered—and it doesn't happen that often anymore, but it did in the early days—at some point I learned that I needed to work on that. So, I would get triggered, and I would own it to the client, which was scary at first because I thought clients would no longer respect me if I talked about the part of me they triggered. But it turned out to be the opposite. They really liked it, as long as I could stay present, as long as I was talking about it from Self. Then, between sessions I would do a piece of work in therapy or supervision with a therapist on the trailhead that had come up in the session. As a result of doing that, as I say, I'm a very different person. There's nothing like working with certain clients to bring up the parts in you that you need to heal. For 20 years I was working with this very traumatized clientele with these terrible diagnoses, and they have both extreme protectors, which will trigger you, and they also have incredibly sensitive parts detectors. So, they can notice your parts very easily, even when you're not aware of them, and if you're lucky, they'll call you out on them. They'll often call you out in an extreme way, and they'll attribute to what you're doing a lot of things that aren't true. So, it's easy to get defensive and try to say, "No, I wasn't doing it for that reason, and why are you being so mean?" But if you don't go there and, instead, you just listen for the kernel of truth in what they say and then apologize, their protectors will usually calm down.

Anyway, that's the long way of saying that that's my philosophy for all of us—that we use our clients as tor-mentors, and when I'm doing super-vision, I'm just trying to help therapists do that.

Supervision and Stuckness Over Time

In the UK, supervision is for life.
  What do you mean?
  Well, even if you're qualified and have been working for 30, 40 years, if you're accredited by certain professional bodies, you are required to have a certain amount of supervision each month.
  Oh, that's very interesting. I don't think that's true here.
  No, and I don't know quite why I said that.
  I can support that. I don't have the same kinds of clients that I used to, and I don't get stuck nearly as often now, so I don't these days feel the need for a lot of supervision. But, if I had that same client caseload, then I certainly would. And, you know, I'm married to a good IFS supervisor. We talk about cases, and we help each other, so I guess supervision is for life for me too.

Knowing which Parts to Go to First

Yes, and over the decades you've acquired a vast amount of experience. Using the example from this week (Schwartz, 2020) with the second supervisee, you were explaining something about your experience with what she called "speed demon" parts, and you were helping with case conceptualization—which parts to go to first.
  Exactly. Yes, so it's not like all I do is work with therapists' parts. I'll also try to give perspective. Also, because when working with many clients, especially trauma survivors, there is a sequence to which parts you can work with first and which you can't, even among protectors.

Pushing Parts

In the example you highlight, there's this big pushing part, and she didn't know—and I didn't know in the beginning—that there are consequences to going to that part first. It seems the pushing, eager part is an ally in the beginning as it just wants to get in there, heal it all, and get out. It's easy to ally with a pushing part, but then all the protectors that are afraid of going too fast feel pressured and dig in their heels, and you'd get polarization of some kind. I wanted to give the supervisee some perspective: "You are kind of siding with that pushing part, and that's why you're having a problem."
  Yes, there are times, for sure, where I'll try to give a big picture about what is happening. I think I remember saying to her that whenever I get wind of a pushing part, that's almost always the part I'll start with, because as long as it's pushing, you'll get the backlash.
  Yes, the polarization. So, Dick, would you mind explaining more about sequences of parts that often come up?

The critic in the addictive triangle

In addictions there's usually a triangle of parts: the addictive part that takes you to the activity; the manager, often a pretty brutal critic, who is trying to control that [first] one; and then there's the exile they are both trying to help. What I've found over and over is if you start with the addictive part, then the critic is jumping in like crazy, but if you start with the critic, then after you've got the critic defused you can go to the addictive part and the work goes a lot more easily. (See Sykes, 2017, 2021; Sykes & Sweezy, 2022)

Suicidal parts

There's a whole series of those little tips that I've learned. Another would be that whenever there's a threatening suicidal part (or any kind of really scary firefighter) lurking around in the system, then all the parts are afraid that if you go anywhere in the system it will trigger that button. The part becomes a limiter, like a regulator in an engine or something, and there's only so much you can do while that bomb is still lurking around waiting to explode. Whenever I get wind of that one, I'll go to that one first and defuse that bomb, and then all the parts relax, and you can do a lot of work. I don't think I've written about this, but there are these patterns that are typical stuck points that therapists who don't know about them get caught up in.

Yes, and beginning therapists might not have experienced working with that pattern of protectors.

Transitioning from other orientations includes losing the fear of certain parts

Yes, or they come from other orientations in which, for example, going to a suicidal part isn't something you would do until you've gone through this whole containment and resourcing first stage. This might involve teaching the client various skills, and you don't go to these scary places until the client seems to not be so fragile. IFS is a totally different orientation.

It is worth emphasizing that there are lots of other psychotherapeutic approaches that lead to therapists being very frightened of certain parts. These approaches don't think of parts as parts but as pathological psychological processes. A key aspect of supervision is pumping the fear out of therapists that was pumped into them by these other approaches and helping them see—that "P word" perspective (see "5 Ps" in the Glossary)—that these are just protective parts, nothing more. If, as a therapist, you aren't afraid of them and you can get your client to not be afraid of them, then you can go to these extreme protectors right away and have that conversation, "What are you afraid would happen if you didn't kill her?" The part will say some version of, "She'd be in pain all the time. I can't stand how much pain she's in." I reply, "Okay, if we could heal that pain would you still have to kill her?" The part comes back with, "No, but I don't think you can do that." I do some hope merchanting, "Would you give us a chance to prove that we can? I guarantee we can."

A lot of therapists don't know to have that conversation or don't have the confidence to make those promises. That's another aspect of my supervision, I'm lending supervisees my confidence.

I'm thinking dissociation is another example of that.

That's another good example, and so many therapists are, "Oh my God, she's dissociating." And I'm, "No, there's this protector jumped in and took her brain." You can do direct access with the dissociating part, and it will tell you why it jumped in most of the time. Then you negotiate with it. So yeah, an important part of supervision is reminding therapists of the basics of the IFS model when they get stuck, because they often get stuck because they go back to their old orientation.

Getting unstuck may involve asking the client's parts

Or, maybe they're not sure about the next stage of the process for some reason.

Sure, especially with a population like the clients we talked about on the Continuity Program this week (Schwartz, 2020). You're going to get stuck. You can't not get stuck with those clients, and it helps to be aware of that. You know, I got stuck all the time with those clients. I would try all kinds of things and not get anywhere, and at some point my managers would step back, and almost out of desperation I would say, "I have no idea what to do now. Does anybody in there know what to do?" And somebody would come out and say, "Do this." The part would tell me, "You've got to go to the suicidal part," and I'd be, "Oh, of course." That's another thing I'm trying to do, free up therapists to let their clients know when they are stuck and collaborate with their clients. A lot of times the client's parts will teach us directly—that's how I learned this model, from my clients.

Yes, from the clients and the wisdom in their parts and their system.

Taking the shame out of getting it wrong

Yeah, and a lot of time their parts were open enough to share with me what I was doing wrong.

Mm hmm, now I'm thinking about working with a supervisee who has parts up around being stuck. There's no shame in being stuck, you've been stuck, I've been stuck, everybody gets stuck.

Yeah, I like to normalize it, and, as I say, you cannot not get stuck with certain clients—there is no shame in asking for help. And, most of the time, there are parts of you involved in being stuck, and there's no shame in that either. In fact, your wisdom and courage at looking at your parts and working with them is to be applauded. That's what I did and why we're here now.

A Turning Point in Practicing Supervision

Dick, is there's anything that stands out in your history of either being a supervisor or being a supervisee that you would like to share? Any memories or stories or turning points for you?

You know, there was a long time when I thought supervision was about telling the therapist what they were doing wrong and what they should do differently. It also paralleled my therapy at the time, which was to tell clients what they were doing wrong and what they should do differently, and it wasn't until—and these are some of the early years, maybe the 90s—I started to get to know and trust Self more and more, my own and the Self of my clients and my supervisees, and I would try increasingly, instead of telling somebody what to do, say "What do you want to do now?" when they were in Self. Increasingly, I was amazed that they knew what to do at all these different levels, and that act is actually quite empowering. A lot of the goal for me is to empower therapists to trust that they actually do have it in them, and they just need to work with their own parts, and the more I tell them what to do, the less they do that.

Yes, the less empowered they feel.

The less empowered they feel, the more they rely on someone like me, and they get stuck. So that's part of the philosophy. I've become a kind of minimalist—it's true that there are a lot of times when I'll give supervisees content and perspective, but I try to minimize it, and I try my best to empower therapists.

Yes, and then that flows down. Like you say, if the therapist is empowered, they can empower the client and the client's system, and they can recall the client has a Self, and the Self is the one we try to give leadership to in the client's system.

It's all parallel that way. If you learned through being lectured at, you're going to do that with yourself, with your parts, and with clients. But if somebody helped you trust your own Self, you're going to help your client trust their own Self.

Role Modeling Has a Place

Yes, and sometimes, it feels like that's it. In a nutshell, you know, "Do we need to talk further?" But also, I guess, part of why I hope this book is going to be interesting is that there are more things supervisors can do. I remember, way back on the Continuity Program, you did a role-play with a supervisee, for example.

Yeah, I'll also try to demonstrate what I would do. It's a bit uncomfortable, but there are a lot of people who talk about WWDD? (playing off WWJD?—in Christian circles, What Would Jesus Do?).

(Laughing) *Ah, What Would Dick Do?!*

And I don't mind that in the beginning. IFS is very counterintuitive compared to a lot of other things, and as therapists struggle to make that transition, they do need to borrow some of my confidence and some of my "in your bones knowledge." It used to bother me as I'm all about empowering people, but there's some necessary degree of role modeling, you know, role-plays are one way to do that. It's also why I show the videos. Role modeling is part of supervision too.

A Lifelong Interest in Supervision

That leads me to think of supervision of supervision, which I also find very helpful, especially as I'm just beginning to be a supervisor of supervisors, so, you know, it goes on all the way up, as it were.

Yeah, supervision has always been a big interest of mine. I was a co-author of a book called *The Handbook of Family Therapy Supervision* (Liddle et al., 1988). This was before IFS. At the same time as I was developing the model, I was in this little family therapy training program, and we used to spend a lot of time talking about supervision. This was back in the day when the one-way mirror was a big thing and had broken onto the scene. We converted a lot of the rooms that way, and we had earphones in the therapist's ear.

With the supervisors talking into them?

Yeah, we did a lot of live supervision, walking in and giving statements to the families at times. Wild days. Anyway, I was one of the authors on this handbook, which is still in print, as far as I know, so it's always been an interest of mine.

IFS Supervision Training

At the moment, there's no one sort of training in supervision anywhere, in the US or the UK.

You mean in IFS?

Yes, there's no official IFS training in supervision.

We are going to launch this year training for trainers, which won't be exactly that but will contain elements of helping trainers be good supervisors.

Great, yes. So that's in 2020.

Yes. It's partly because becoming an IFS lead trainer is a long marathon in itself, and with the demand now we just don't have enough trainers, so we're finding ways to expedite that journey. The training for trainers can help people skip a couple of years, I'm hoping.

The Value of IFS Group Supervision

Okay. Have you ever done any group supervision for IFS?

Yes, I just ended a telegroup on the phone that I had run for many years—the same group basically, with a few people coming and going. I think there were 12 or 13 people. Each session was once a month for two hours, and maybe four or five different people—sort of like the Continuity Program—would present a case, and I'd wind up, again, 70 percent of the time working with their parts. That group I only ended because I was just overwhelmed. I really enjoyed it, and the group got incredibly close. They would reconnect at the conference every year, and I found it very enjoyable. So yeah, it's very possible to do it in a group context. As people listen to each other and where they're getting stuck, and then they listen to the parts that they work with, just like in the trainings, they feel very connected to the supervisee doing the work and give them a lot of support, and they are also learning about their own parts and how they get stuck with clients too.

I guess that's another thing, especially at these times, part of my philosophy of supervision is about connection and helping somebody not feel alone with stuff, so a group like that, I can understand how it might get really close and supportive and be really valuable.

Yeah, I felt terrible ending it because people were so upset. Now that I sit around the house, I could probably do it. At the time when we ended, my life was getting too far out of control.

Yeah, that was a good question, I can't think of any other topics.

No? Great. Shall we end it there?

Sounds good.

March 29, 2020

References

Liddle, H. A., Breunlin, C. D., & Schwartz, R. C. (1988). *The handbook of family therapy supervision.* The Guilford Press.

Schwartz, R. C. (2020, March 26). Month 3 call with Richard Schwartz in IFS Continuity Program [Webinar]. In N. Sowell & R. C. Schwartz, *IFS treatment for healing and restoring health: Freedom from trauma, early adversity, and toxic stress affecting the mind and body* [Online Course]. IFS Institute.

Sykes, C. (2017). An IFS lens on addiction: Compassion for extreme parts. In M. Sweezy & E. L. Ziskind (Eds.), *Innovations and elaborations in Internal Family Systems therapy* (pp. 29–48). Routledge.

Sykes, C. (2021, February 01). "Polarization: The battlefield" in IFS continuity program month 2 Compassion for addictive processes [Webinar]. In R. C. Schwartz, C. Sykes, & F. G. Anderson, *Trauma and the addictive process, an IFS lens* [Online Course]. IFS Institute.

Sykes, C., & Sweezy, M. (2022). *Internal Family Systems: A strengths-based approach to addictive process.* PESI, forthcoming.

2 A Model of IFS-Informed Supervision and Consultation

Unblending from Struggle into Self-Led Clarity

Dan Reed and Ray Wooten

IFS-Informed Supervision Overture

The supervisor is in a unique position as the etymology of the word from the Medieval Latin verb *supervidere*, meaning to "oversee", connotes. Since the late 1970s, supervision has been developing as its own discipline, recognized as a primary method for teaching and supporting novice and experienced counselors (Borders & Brown, 2005; Holloway, 1995). As the field of supervision has developed within the field of psychotherapy, it has become clear that despite similarities, supervision is not synonymous with counseling. Specialized training in supervision is both useful and often necessary on the path to becoming a competent supervisor (Borders, 1992).

Specific training is invaluable to orient a supervisor, who may find themselves working with therapists ranging from beginner to advanced. Helping any therapist learn a new perspective and model of change can be challenging. Since exposure to and training in the Internal Family Systems (IFS) model of psychotherapy most often occurs post-graduation, those offering supervision or consultation informed by IFS will often work with therapists more experienced in non-IFS modalities. Supervision training can help orient a supervisor supporting such therapists, remembering that expert therapists, like everyone else, become beginners while learning something new.

This chapter outlines and describes a model of supervision and consultation that integrates IFS into the process of supervision. We refer to this model as IFS-informed consultation. It serves as a framework for orienting and training supervisors and consultants already trained in or curious about IFS. This process of supervision is relevant for supporting therapists learning the IFS model of psychotherapy as well as for therapists working within any other model of psychotherapy. For those readers who are already experienced supervisors and consultants utilizing IFS in their practice, we trust that reading this chapter will affirm your current practices and/or offer a reflective resource with which to dialogue. The material is based on doctoral research by Reed (2019), a summary of which is included at the end of the chapter and may be of particular use to new consultants or consultants new to IFS.

DOI: 10.4324/9781003044864-2

For the purposes of this chapter, the authors lean on a vision of supervision created by Hawkins and Shohet (with contributions from Ryde and Wilmot) (2012, p. 60), which states:

> Supervision is a joint endeavor in which a practitioner with the help of a supervisor, attends to their clients, themselves as part of their client practitioner relationships and the wider systemic context, and by so doing improves the quality of their work, transforms their client relationships, continuously develops themselves, their practice and the wider profession.

This foundational definition of supervision underscores a process of simultaneously attending to the multiple layers of internal and external relationships that continually interact and impact the supervisory process, which weaves nicely with an IFS perspective.

To highlight the collaborative process of IFS-informed consultation, we have chosen the terms *consultation/consultant* to refer to the processes of both supervision and consultation. The term *therapist* will be used in place of supervisee/consultee. The choice of these terms is intended to help the writers and readers step out of the North American language/meaning of the term *supervision*, as applying only to a process carried out by an external authority with power over pre-licensed, subordinate, and developing supervisees, with the burdens and constrictions within that structure. We advocate that a change in language will promote a more universal lens that views consultation as part of a psychotherapist's lifelong development.

Overview of the Key Features of IFS-Informed Consultation

IFS-informed consultation shares the general goals for supervision that Hawkins and Shohet (2012) describe above. However, the process of IFS-informed consultation offers specific elements that increase possibilities for relational collaboration, consultant transparency, and therapist empowerment. These elements include the foundational IFS principles of Self-leadership, multiplicity of mind, and systems thinking. Additional elements within IFS-informed consultation include processes for working relationally, both internally and externally; explicit contracting and recontracting within a session; learning and exploring experientially; unblending; and the role of the consultant.

These foundational and process elements combine to create an atmosphere to collaboratively support therapists in developing their embodied experience and awareness of reciprocal Self–part relating. These elements also foster the therapist's ability to check the present moment and assess their own and their client's level of Self-leadership based on internal and external experiential markers (see Table 2.1 below). IFS-informed consultation provides opportunities for therapists to experience the possibility and freedom of being a professional who is in relationship with and informed by their parts (i.e., Self-led).

Before describing the full structure of our model of IFS-informed consultation, we review the concepts of Self-leadership, multiplicity of mind, unblending, the role of a consultant, and the intention of consultation. Within an IFS-informed consultation process, everyone (i.e., consultant, psychotherapist, client) is actively involved in the process of recognizing and developing Self-leadership. Self-leadership is a present-moment experience of being in relationship with, informed by, and advocating for one's parts. Rather than thinking of a person as having a unitary mind and singular ways of thinking and being, people using the IFS model recognize that all of us have multiple competing drives happening simultaneously. Within this way of conceptualizing the mind, the term *parts* is used as a shorthand way of differentiating aspects of our experience that have their own consistent range of thoughts, feelings, sensations, and impulses for movement/action. For therapists, some common parts-related experiences that impact their professional life include feeling anxious, inadequate, incompetent, and overwhelmed; wanting to be seen as competent; and feeling over responsible for themselves and their clients.

This experience of parts interacting directly with the world is what people in the IFS world call "being blended with parts" or "being driven by parts." Trouble can ensue when therapists unwittingly do therapy or "act out" from these states. Meanwhile, *unblending* is a process of differentiating from one's parts and getting into relationship with those parts. In other words, unblending is the process by which a person increases their level of Self-leadership.

A consultant utilizing the IFS model to support and inform the consultation process has some unique ways of being, which place them in more intimate relationship with themselves and the therapists they work with than may be common within consultation/supervision at large. For instance, a primary way of teaching within an IFS-informed consultation process is through direct and explicit experience with the IFS process. As such, the consultant embodies and models the IFS way of being, sharing their Self presence with the therapists they work with. This sharing offers needed containment for understandably anxious parts of therapists, especially those who are in the midst of learning a new way of being and working with clients with very real and sometimes frightening struggles.

While Self-led, the consultant models their present-moment relationship with their own parts and their awareness of the therapist and the therapist's parts. The IFS-informed consultant contracts explicitly to be the *parts detector* for themselves, the therapist they are working with, and the therapist's client. As a parts detector, the consultant takes on the responsibility of noticing parts and making explicit invitations for the therapist to be in more direct relationship with their own parts, become curious about their client's parts, and sometimes share some of their own present-moment awareness of their own parts or ways their parts have behaved in psychotherapy, for better and for worse. Simultaneously, the consultant invites and welcomes the therapist to notice and inquire about the presence of the consultant's parts within their process together. In this way, the consultant's fallibility is on the table and part of the discussion, humanizing the process and increasing the possibility for reduced hierarchy and a more relational experience for all involved. Throughout, the consultant leans on the structure and language of the IFS process and its ongoing invitations into experience, modeling the IFS process for the therapist. Through directly experiencing the IFS model, therapists have the possibility of developing their conceptual understanding and also having a genuine felt sense of supporting and developing reciprocal Self–part relationships to utilize with themselves and with their clients within psychotherapy.

The most significant difference between IFS as it is applied to psychotherapy and consultation is the intention. Though the goals and form may at times appear identical, psychotherapy seeks to support a person's development, well-being, and healing in all areas of life, whereas consultation seeks to support a professional's development toward increased effectiveness within their psychotherapy practice. For the consultant–therapist contract, the extent to which it supports professional development and the professional efficacy of the therapist within the realm of psychotherapy defines the consultation process. Everything explored or supported in IFS-informed consultation is specifically related back to the therapist's clinical work and development as a professional.

Flow of the Model

IFS-informed consultation has a general contract for the trajectory of consultation, which is collaboratively negotiated between the consultant and the therapist in the beginning (Reed, 2019). This agreement has a focus on the development of the therapist to co-create effective psychotherapeutic outcomes for their clients. It explores the:

- Format of consultation (individual or group, frequency, duration, fee, etc.);
- The therapist's wishes and goals for seeking consultation (to explore therapist parts, unblending, achieve IFS certification, focus on a particular client, increase general IFS competence or competence in general, for practice, etc.); and
- The consultant's preferred ways of working (role-play, recordings, case presentation, skills focus, U-turning, direct teaching, etc.).

This initial agreement for the scope of consultation may or may not include an explicit discussion of how exiles will be worked with or how trailheads will be marked for exploring within consultation or elsewhere. However, these specifics will form part of the ongoing recontracting within sessions and from session to session.

Figure 2.1 shows the non-linear, cycling process from a consultant's perspective, where a consultant and a therapist collaboratively work together in a consultation session. This framework applies most directly to working with an individual but can readily be applied with a consultation group.

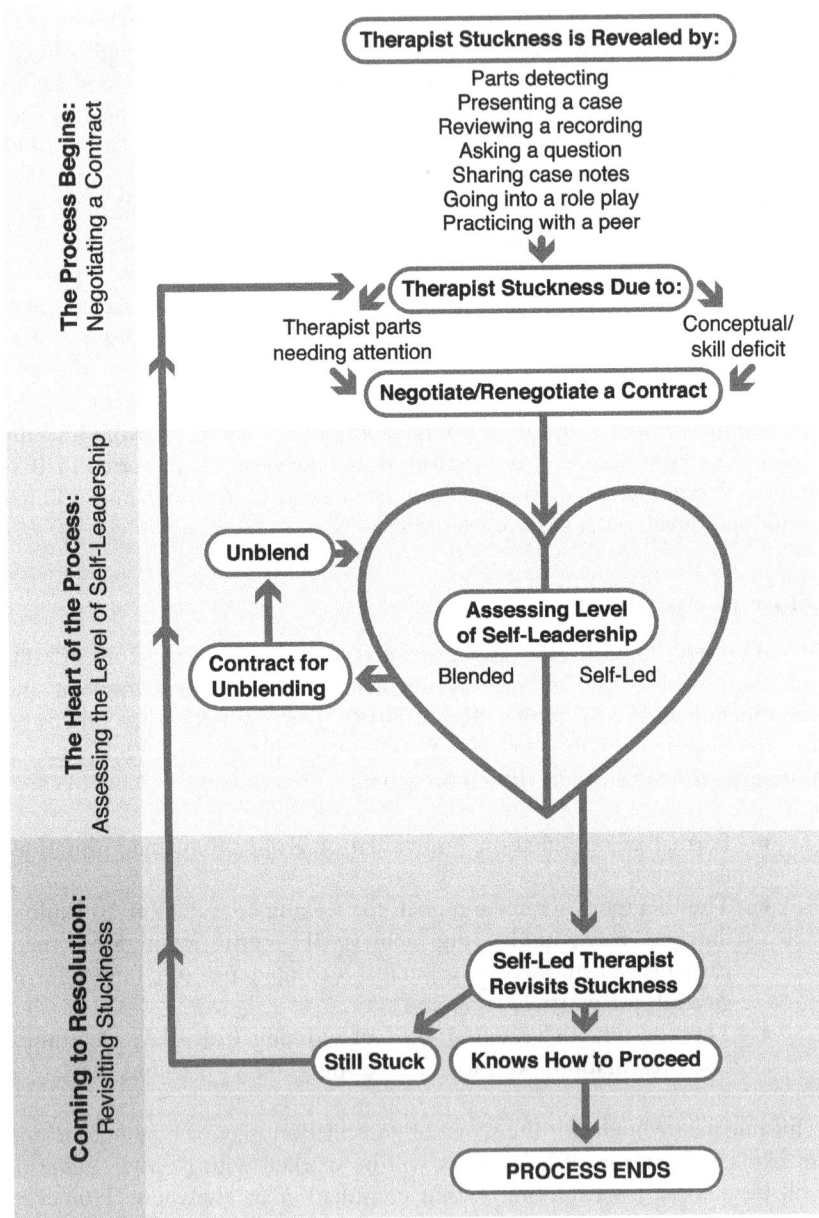

Figure 2.1 The Flow of IFS-Informed Consultation

Unlike other models of supervision, in which a hierarchy is important and an unhelpful imbalance of power can occur, in an IFS-informed process the consultant and therapist both agree to continuously monitor their own and each other's level of Self-leadership while inviting open inquiry into the other's level of Self-leadership. The consultant contracts to take the lead in assessing the level of Self-leadership within the consultation process while sharing this responsibility with the therapist or therapists. The intention is for therapists to develop greater and greater sensitivity to their and any other's level of Self-leadership.

To summarize the flow of individual consultation sessions diagrammed in Figure 2.1, the three-phased process begins by collaboratively negotiating a contract around the therapist's stuckness. It continues to the consultant and the therapist assessing the therapist's level of Self-leadership and (as needed) supporting the therapist unblending to a point where both the consultant and therapist sense the therapist is sufficiently Self-led. Once the therapist experiences this greater level of differentiation with their parts, the consultant and therapist **revisit** the therapist's stuckness in relation to the presenting problem. In this final step of revisiting the therapist's stuckness, the consultant and therapist get a sense of the therapist's level of Self-leadership, and whether the therapist knows what to do (or not) determines whether the iterative cycle continues to further increase the therapist's level of Self-leadership in relation to themselves and their client, or whether it shifts into teaching a skill or concept that the therapist may need.

The Process Begins: Negotiating a Contract (Phase 1)

While negotiating the contract, the consultant and therapist collaboratively sort out what they will explore and how they might explore that for the session. The contract within IFS-informed consultation is created to move toward resolution of the therapist's feelings of stuckness concerning a particular client or a concept or skill so that the therapist can re-engage within their therapy relationship(s) to feel more confident in their ability to be effective. In the process of identifying the therapist's stuckness, the consultant and therapist collaborate to ascertain whether the stuckness feels more like a part or parts clouding a therapist's abilities or an actual skill deficit, which may or may not create a cloud of parts.

The therapist's stuckness may be revealed in different ways: through the therapist presenting a case, sharing a recording of their work, asking a question, sharing case notes, going into a role-play, or, if in a group, doing a practice session with another therapist and getting live support from the consultant. Regardless of the path in, the consultant contracts to act as a parts detector, watching, listening, and sensing for the therapist's parts and level of Self-leadership as well as their own. Through watching, sensing, and listening together, the consultant seeks to form an explicit agreement regarding their intention for the session.

Anything interfering with the therapist's efficacy as a therapist is grist for the mill in this process, but for this discussion let us consider something fairly common within consultation: the therapist blaming their client for the stuckness in therapy. A therapist practicing IFS might begin consultation by saying, "The client just doesn't have enough Self-energy. I'm tired of providing all of the Self-energy every session and dealing with all of their protectors." Whereas a therapist trained in another therapeutic modality might say, "The client just doesn't care. I'm not even sure they want to be in therapy. I'm tired of working harder than my client." In the background, even if it's not said explicitly, the consultant can hear that part or parts of the therapist feel inadequate as a therapist.

The consultant continues contracting by either offering the therapist a possibility for what and how they might explore for the session or accepting a request from the therapist regarding something they would like some support around. In the above example of a therapist feeling the burden of carrying the load for their client, the consultant can offer the therapist a variety of ways to work with their stuckness:

U-Turning

"What if we could help you feel like you have some more options, whether your client changes anything they're doing or not?"

"What if we could help get the part of you that's efforting some support so they don't have to work so hard and maybe even get to feel better about where the therapy is at?"

Watching/Listening to a Recording

"Maybe we could look at the video from your last session with this client so that you can show me what's happening, and you can describe more about what you're seeing, thinking, sensing, and intending for you and for them."

Role-Play/Live Practice

"How would you feel about taking on the role of your client and really being them as I take on the role of the therapist? Maybe then you could get a feel both for what it's like being them in general and sense how some interventions might feel from their perspective?"

Therapist Self-Report/Case Presentation

"Maybe you could tell me more about your client, the case, what you've been trying, and what support you'd like from me."

Teaching/Learning

"It sounds like you could use some support just conceptualizing this case, what might be normal for clients like this, and some ways you might work to get a bit more traction. Would you like to hear me talk about this for a little while, or is there something else you're looking for?"

No matter which invitation is contracted for or renegotiated along the way, the intention of consultation remains the same:

- Support the therapist in unblending so they can become more Self-led in relationship with themselves and their client(s);
- Strengthen the therapist's ability to track evidence for a person's level of Self-leadership in themselves and others;
- Develop the therapist's skill of present-moment Self–part relating within themselves (and facilitating that in others); and
- Teach the therapist concepts and skills they may need.

The Heart of the Process: Assessing the Level of Self-Leadership (Phase 2)

The authors intentionally placed assessing the therapist's level of Self-leadership in the center of the diagram of the flow of IFS-informed consultation. This phase consists of the consultant continuously tracking and inquiring into the therapist's level of Self-leadership, which serves as the central piece of the consultation work. The goal of the consultatory exploration and instruction is to enhance the 5 Ps of the therapist (perspective, presence, playfulness, persistence, and patience), while uncovering more of the 8 Cs, qualities that point to the presence of Self (confidence, courage, clarity, compassion, curiosity, creativity, calm, and connectedness) in the face of their stuckness (Reed, 2019; Schwartz, 2013; Schwartz & Sweezy, 2020). The guiding belief is that through unblending from parts, the therapist will increase their level of Self-leadership and experience an affective shift, which may allow them to reflect on their situation with a client with more confidence and clarity in how to be with themselves and their client. Meanwhile, as the therapist unblends, it may become clearer to both the consultant and therapist that the therapist doesn't know what do. In that case, the consultant can support the therapist in developing skills and/or conceptual understandings as needed.

In this model of IFS-informed consultation, the consultant and therapist contract for unblending for as long as the therapist feels stuck and lacks a critical mass of the 5 Ps and 8 Cs. Choosing the method for unblending, whether doing a U-turn, watching/listening to a recording, role-play/live practice, therapist self-report, or teaching, is part of the initial contract and ongoing recontracting. The consultant also respects when the therapist decides they have gone as far as they wish to for the moment. Since the whole process is collaborative, recontracting explicitly at each next step along the way plays a crucial role in supporting collaboration and the therapist's sense of safety. Recontracting may include:

- Shifting the focus of investigation;
- Checking if the current or next level of depth/vulnerability is okay for the therapist (for example, getting to know a part, unblending, making contact with an exile, witnessing an exile, or unburdening an exile);
- Truncating the process prior to resolution;
- Marking a trailhead to explore in their own therapy or elsewhere; or
- Shifting methods for the therapist to complete their unblending process with the consultant (for example, role-play/live practice, video, teaching, U-turn, or self-report).

Within the contracting process, the consultant and therapist choose methods for unblending to match the therapist's current openness to being vulnerable within consultation. On the end of the spectrum of methods of unblending where the therapist is most likely to feel vulnerable, there is the U-turn: bringing the attention directly to the therapist and their parts in the struggle with their client. U-turning is an opportunity for developing the experiential skill of reciprocal Self–part relating, resulting in Self-regulation. On the other end of the spectrum of unblending methods likely to create the least vulnerable feelings for the therapist, there is unblending through teaching or skill building (for example, a consultant teaching when in-sight, direct access, and externalizing are useful and what each looks like). Teaching and skill building can slow down and soothe some therapist parts by either confirming and affirming what parts know or filling in a needed conceptual gap or skills deficit. This potentially less activating or personally revealing approach offers a therapist's parts co-regulation.

Tracking for Self-Leadership

Tracking is the skill the consultant utilizes and models for the therapist, inviting the therapist to continually develop and join in with the consultant so that together they may assess the therapist's (and consultant's) level of Self-leadership (see Table 2.1).

Possible process markers that point toward the therapist having reached a Self-led threshold in consultation include:

- The therapist is in relationship with initially activated parts, forming a Self-led team of parts.
- The parts that had been activated in relation to the presenting situation (i.e., stuckness) are aware of the therapist.
- The therapist and their parts have developed a relationship where the therapist sees, hears, and/or senses the parts that were trying to help in therapy, and the parts that were trying to help in therapy sense the

Table 2.1 Markers Used to Track Level of Self-Leadership

Voice tone/prosody/timbre	Is the voice quality lower or higher, rhythmic or clipped, rich or terse?
Body tension	Check jaw, shoulders, forehead: are they softer or more contracted?
Posture	Check for soft stability as compared to rigidity or collapse.
Movement/impulses to move	Check for level of directed, relaxed, free, completed movement compared to repetitive, intense, restrained, incomplete movement.
Breath	Notice the breath pattern: is it deeper and slower, shallow and quick, or holding?
Word choice	Listen to the language: is it openly descriptive or laced with judgment?
Speaking	*For* the experience (of a part) rather than *from* the experience (as that part).
Eyes	Notice the gaze: is it soft and steady or concentrated and narrow?
Response from others	Notice the impact on others: do they become more receptive or more closed off, avoidant, or combative?
Energy consumption	Notice whether a way of being/doing is energy giving or draining.

Source: Adapted from Dubin and Stewart, 2017

presence of the therapist and feel seen, heard, and/or sensed from their perspective.

- The parts that have contributions for therapy and want to participate in therapy have been explicitly invited to be part of the team with the therapist in session and feel welcomed and included. Those that don't want to contribute are aware that they are welcome to do something they'd rather be doing for that time.

Note that the integration of the therapist's Self with their parts, as described above, is a goal for consultation rather than healing of the therapist's parts and system.

Markers that indicate exiles feel supported and safe enough, which aids the therapist reaching a Self-led threshold, include:

- Vulnerable parts that felt like they had to stick around during therapy sessions have had some contact with the therapist.
- The therapist and vulnerable part(s) have talked about what the vulnerable one really wants to do while the therapist is in session or at work and have come to some agreement how that can happen.

For example, a five-year-old part of the therapist, who feels scared or overly responsible for a client, can be outside playing when the therapist is in session. The therapist and the young part could have a specific plan for how that will happen. The plan could consist of the therapist chatting with the five-year-old and reminding him/her/it/them where the therapist will be going and inviting the young part to go off and play. The plan could close with the five-year-old and the therapist checking in after the session/work.

Coming to Resolution: Revisiting Stuckness (Phase 3)

Once it appears to the consultant that the therapist has reached a critical mass of Self-leadership, the consultant invites the therapist to sense into their present-moment experience to see how they feel they are doing now. If the therapist reports feeling Self-led and describes some of their present-moment evidence for this (see Table 2.1), then the process moves on to revisit the therapist's stuckness as revealed at the start of the session. However, if the consultant and therapist assess that more unblending would be useful then the process moves back to unblending until both the therapist and consultant agree the therapist has reached a Self-led threshold.

Revisiting stuckness using an internal meditative/imaginative process occurs in both group and individual consultation settings. To do this the consultant makes an invitation saying: "As you consider your client and your situation with them now, what do you notice?" From this invitation, the therapist tracks themselves, their perception of their client, and their sense of the therapist–client relationship (for example, "Notice how you feel toward your client now"). This step may highlight the need for more unblending and affirming Self-leadership or a solid verification of Self-leadership. If the therapist's report and consultant's tracking point toward the therapist being Self-led, then the consultant asks if the therapist knows what to do and/or how to be with the client now. For example, the consultant might say, "From this place and how you're doing now, say more about what you might do or how you might be with your client now."

Once the therapist is Self-led and has a clear sense of the next steps for them and their client, the process of consultation has come to its natural conclusion. If the therapist is Self-led and doesn't "know what to do," then the therapist is primed for teaching. However, if in revisiting the stuckness the therapist still feels stuck (i.e., blended and doesn't know what to do), then the consultation cycle goes back to the beginning. The consultant–therapist team identify the stuckness and recontract for how they might address it. Recontracting and coming to a resolution where the therapist is Self-led and has a clear sense of their next steps may take as little as 30 seconds or may require multiple consultation sessions. Regardless, the cycle continues until the therapist feels Self-led and knows what to do and how to be with their client. To further verify the therapist's embodiment of the 5 Ps and 8 Cs in relation to their initial stuckness, in the following session the consultant can check in with the therapist on how things are actually going with the therapist's client and/or their professional development.

Best Practices of an IFS-Informed Consultant

In this section we summarize what the skilled IFS-informed consultant does within IFS-informed consultation. This section describes some ways in which the consultant models the IFS way of being in relationship with one's Self and others.

Monitoring the Skills of the Therapist

The consultant supports the therapist's development, confidence, and competence. Though the consultant is concerned for the client and has an eye on the client's well-being, the primary focus of the IFS-informed consultant is the therapist's process and skill development. The major skills tracked by the consultant include: (a) assessing one's own and another's level of Self-leadership through tracking, (b) developing one's own Self–part reciprocal relating, (c) facilitating Self–part relating of others, and (d) conceptualizing and being with clients in general and in particularly challenging cases (for example, suicidality, addictive/compulsive processes, dissociative identity disorder, Self-like parts, or those coming with a label of borderline personality disorder).

Co-Creating Safety

The IFS-informed consultant co-creates safety with therapists. Supporting safety begins with the consultant's willingness and ability to be vulnerable and let the therapist behind the curtain a bit. For instance, to support the normalizing of parts and parts reactivity, the consultant may speak of their parts as they have shown up in client sessions through sharing stories and speaking for their parts in the present moment with the therapist. The IFS-informed consultant also invites the therapist to ask the consultant to check in with their parts if the therapist senses something within the present moment that leads the therapist to wonder whether the consultant is currently Self-led.

A major element within the consultation relationship that ensures safety is respecting the consultation contract. Part of respecting the consultation contract includes continually recontracting in the here and now in order to explicitly ensure that the therapist is okay with the present level of internal depth rather than just going along with what the consultant thinks is best (for example, "Is it okay to sense that 5-year-old's presence here with you now?"). Recontracting continues to explicitly address any steps that might move things even further along the internal path (for example, "Maybe we could stay with that five-year-old for just a little bit longer to help him get what he needs so he doesn't have to feel responsible for doing the therapy."). Part of the contract is that the consultant and therapist will assess the level of vulnerability and honor the therapist's process by continually checking in and respecting when and where the therapist's protectors say "Enough."

Contracting

The consultant collaboratively contracts with the therapist, making explicit agreements that seek to support the therapist's development toward greater effectiveness as a therapist. For example:

CONSULTANT: "Maybe we could spend some time with the part of you who's having such a strong reaction to your client."
THERAPIST: "Sure. That would be good."

Tracking/Assessing Level of Self-Leadership

The IFS-informed consultant monitors their own present-moment experience (i.e., thoughts, feelings, sensations, and impulses to move) as well as that of the therapist, observing and becoming curious about both verbal and non-verbal cues. Tracking and inviting relationship with present-moment experience is the process that offers a pathway for the non-conscious and unconscious roles of parts to become conscious. The consultant (and in time the therapist) tracks the nature of present-moment experience using the markers described in Table 2.1.

Recontracting

As noted above, part of what creates safety within IFS-informed consultation is the ongoing, overt recontracting. The consultant extends invitations to confirm whether the direction the process is on feels okay to the therapist, adjusting and calibrating to what feels acceptable to the therapist. This is a collaborative process of getting permission at each step along the way rather than coercing the therapist down a particular path the consultant chooses. In IFS-informed consultation, the therapist's right to privacy is respected by both parties, perhaps more so than in psychotherapy, where there is an expectation of vulnerability on the part of the person coming to the other for a service.

Supporting Unblending

Unblending is a process of supporting a person's parts and increasing Self-leadership within that person. In this process, the Self and part(s) of a person increase both their differentiation and connection. Unblending can happen through either the consultant or therapist relating directly with the activated parts or indirectly through an experience where parts get some of their needs met (for example, the consultant teaching, the therapist talking about something, or the blended person exploring/allowing movement in their body). See the Appendix for descriptions of a wide variety of methods for unblending.

A Summary of the Research: Crucial Concepts of IFS-Informed Consultation for New Consultants and Consultants New to IFS

The Importance of Contracting

Contracting is one of the most crucial elements creating clarity and a safe container for consultation and psychotherapy informed by IFS. In a consulting situation, the consultant contracts to be a parts detector, tracking the therapist and themselves. The consultant continually monitors their own and the therapist's level of Self-leadership as they facilitate movement through stuckness, inviting unblending as needed. The therapist plays a parallel function with their client. A guiding belief within the IFS framework is that "When you encounter a problem in IFS therapy, it is usually because a part is interfering, but you don't know whose it is—the client's or yours." (Schwartz, 1995, p. 88) Consultation offers a place for therapists to get the needs of the parts that show up in their psychotherapy practice met, so that their Self can be more available for their own parts and their clients.

Since consultation is a professional relationship in support of a therapist's professional life, *recontracting* (i.e., ongoing contracting) throughout the session is different than in psychotherapy. In consultation, the therapist's right to privacy is respected even more than in psychotherapy. The consultant will detect parts, but the depth of exploring a therapist's parts and supporting the therapist's relationship with their parts is an ongoing negotiation between the consultant and the therapist. The therapist has the right to mark a trailhead to explore in the future with a therapist or in some other way; to receive support unblending from a part in relation to a client; or, if the consultant and therapist are both open to it and there is time, to work with exiles together. If the consultant believes the therapist's personal material is impacting the therapist's professional ability/competence/development, and if either the consultant suggests or the therapist chooses to address that material elsewhere, then the consultant needs to follow up with the therapist to see how addressing that is progressing. Meanwhile, when parts exploration is happening in consultation, the consultant continually checks implicitly *and* explicitly for the therapist's comfort with the current level of depth, wish for further support, or sense that "this feels like enough for now."

Self-Leadership is a Key Goal for IFS-Informed Consultation

Developing therapist Self-leadership and parts' trust in that Self-leadership is a primary goal of IFS-informed processes. IFS-informed consultation is a place where a therapist can experientially develop the skills of assessing their own and their client's present-moment level of Self-leadership and the skills for developing and fostering inner relationship between a person and their parts. From an IFS perspective, developing these skills to support and embody Self-leadership allows for more effective therapy. The Self-led therapist has more access to what they know as well as more confidence, curiosity, creativity, and courage for stepping into the unknown with their client.

From a Self-led position, parts of the therapist can trust that the therapist's Self is not the only Self available. The Self-led therapist knows that the client's Self is available as well. It is part of the therapist's job to support the client's system in allowing more and more of the client's Self to be present and lead. Self-led awareness opens up possibilities and choice, where a narrowed parts-led position creates an experience of more limited options. Parts-led positions regularly lead to more effortful, coercive interventions by the therapist. Furthermore, the Self-led therapist has people to lean on when stuckness inevitably arises within their work. Colleagues, mentors, their own therapist, and their supervisor or consultant remain resources for reflecting, honing skills, and learning information.

Since the level of a person's Self-leadership is dynamic and varies, tracking the level of Self-leadership and unblending are the primary skills supported and developed within supervision and consultation informed by IFS. Through unblending the goal is always to support parts so that they can relax and increase the therapist's level of Self-leadership. This goal holds for:

- Utilizing a U-turn;
- Collaboratively joining to share responses to a therapist's recording of a therapy session and wondering about choice points and skill application;
- Engaging in a connecting teaching piece;
- Role-playing; or
- Applying any of the other methods for unblending described earlier in this chapter and in the Appendix.

This experiential learning process supports the therapist in developing procedural pathways for finding their way back to Self-leadership from being blended, which is inevitable. Therapists use IFS-informed consultation to develop ways to notice when blending happens in the moment and then to unblend before, during, and after sessions. This level of Self-awareness makes the therapist a better parts detector, for themselves and their clients, giving them a greater ability to support others (i.e., clients) in unblending and developing their own reciprocal Self–part relationships within themselves.

Trust in one's own Self-leadership is the IFS model's path toward that individual's Self-regulation. Self-regulation is a state of experiencing less reactivity from one's parts and more harmony among them, while still offering parts a way to get their needs met. Developing confidence and skill in gaining and restoring Self-leadership through experiences in consultation is a crucial element within the IFS-informed way of improving the efficacy of the therapist's work with their clients.

An IFS-Informed Consultation Framework

As depicted by a grounded theory study I (DR) conducted in 2018, IFS-informed consultation in the US is typically, though not exclusively, performed with therapists who are licensed professionals wanting to apply the IFS model of psychotherapy within their work with clients (Reed, 2019). The majority of the IFS-informed consultants I interviewed worked primarily with therapists who have done a Level 1 IFS training, though some applied IFS-informed supervision in agency, university, and private practice settings with therapists practicing other models of psychotherapy and who were not seeking IFS training. For those wishing to learn the IFS process, IFS consultants reported that IFS trainings expedite the therapist's development within IFS and allow them to be ready to deepen their process through consultation rather than trying to learn all aspects of IFS over an indefinite period of time within consultation.

The research revealed IFS-informed consultation being practiced individually and in groups as well as in person and via teleconference or videoconference. Due to the highly experiential methods of learning within this model, group consultation offers the greatest range of possibilities for methods of teaching and practicing and developing a peer group. Groups offer therapists a supportive peer network in which the experience of parts can be normalized. Meanwhile, individual consultation offers the advantage of greater flexibility of scheduling and also allows the individual therapist to get more targeted support from their consultant.

For those interviewed, the methods for doing consultation relied primarily on self-report (i.e., case presentation), role-play, direct teaching, and, for some consultants, recordings. Throughout each of these methods the consultant acts as a parts detector, assessing the level of Self-leadership of the therapist and collaboratively checking in with the therapist's experience of themselves to verify whether unblending may be useful and/or wanted. The consultation contract is to support the therapist with their effectiveness with clients and their development as a therapist. To ensure this contract remains explicit, the consultant recontracts continuously for present-moment agreement regarding what they are exploring, how they will do this, and the level to which parts are directly supported within the process (i.e., marking trailheads, unblending from protectors, or witnessing and unburdening exiles).

Case presentation, role-plays, and live practice offer opportunities for live consultation and experiential learning around stuck places. These interactive experiential processes are used to invite and encourage the therapist's struggle to surface, so that it may be explored in real time. These IFS-informed experiential formats sidestep the valid concern that self-reporting provides an edited version of reality, whereby the therapist's protectors manage their anxiety and image. What is less known in the self-reporting process is how the therapist's client is actually presenting the client's unedited wishes and views of their circumstances.

Though it is possible for teaching to become a part-driven, all-knowing supervisor event, that is not how it needs to play out. Within IFS-informed consultation, teaching can be a collaborative way of unblending and/or educating parts. Teaching can be a way for the consultant to speak directly to a part of the therapist and address its fear(s). It can also be a process whereby the consultant supports a therapist's parts by creating a conceptual or skill bridge that helps something make sense to the therapist so their parts can relax. Teaching can offer context to normalize an experience, and, perhaps most importantly and most often in this collaborative process, the therapist can request for the consultant to teach on a particular topic, concept, skill, or context.

Being Self-led is not always enough for a therapist to know what to do. Sometimes a therapist can be in a Self-led state and lack confidence and ability because they are missing some important information about the IFS model, a way of being, or an application within a particular context. Spending time in consultation developing a conceptual map or a skill can be exactly what is needed for the therapist to slide from stuckness into a confident Self-led state with open curiosity in relation to their client. For this reason, the IFS-informed consultant continuously asks in the back of their mind, "Unblending? Skills? Concepts?" A nice thing about working informed by an IFS perspective is that the consultant doesn't need to *know* the ultimate answer—all they need to do is ask. Continuously. And they need to be open to the feedback from the therapist and the therapist's parts.

According to the research, a less widely used method within IFS-informed consultation was incorporating recordings. Recordings can be invaluable for noticing parts' behaviors, for identifying skills that could benefit from honing or choice points that could be explored, and for getting unedited feedback of the efficacy of therapist's work with clients. For working with recordings within IFS-informed consultation, the authors recommend utilizing interpersonal process recall (IPR) (Kagan & Kagan, 1997), though none of the consultants interviewed mentioned this process. IPR is similar to the U-turn in that instead of watching the recording and wondering what is going on for the client, the therapist turns their attention toward themselves and what may be at play within their process. In other words, the consultant encourages the therapist to describe their underlying thoughts and feelings while watching video playback. In essence, the therapist is asked to blend with and/or notice the parts activated within the recorded session—get to know the parts' perspectives and what those parts were attempting to do in the session as well as how those parts view or viewed the therapist, the client, and the situation as it unfolded.

Some of the reasons the American consultants who were interviewed gave for shying away from using recordings include: consultant discomfort with the technological learning that may be involved to work with a recording via video conference, therapist worry about introducing the client to the idea of recording sessions, or the perceived/actual time and money investment required by the consultant and/or therapist to review the recorded material. In other countries, outside influences can create significant barriers to utilizing recording. Complexities around general data protection regulation (GDPR) and professional bodies' client confidentiality codes can inhibit consultants from using recording as a source of information and professional development.

Closing Thoughts

IFS-informed consultation offers the possibility for the consultants and therapists to collaborate and empower everyone in the process. We all need spaces where we can drop appearances of everything being fine and wade into the very real struggles we all face in being with ourselves and others in psychotherapy. Consultation can be that place for therapists. Wherever we are in our ongoing learning trajectories as professionals and human beings, the IFS model and processes offer us a container to support us in being who we really are and feeling what we are actually feeling. It enables us to show up more fully and relationally with ourselves and those with whom we interact.

References

Borders, D. (1992). Learning to think like a supervisor. *The Clinical Supervisor, 10*(2), 135–148.

Borders, D., & Brown, L. (2005). *The new handbook of counseling supervision.* Routledge.

Dubin, R., & Stewart, S. (2017). *Checklist for noticing blending.* Unpublished manuscript.

Hawkins, P., & Shohet, R. (2012). *Supervision in the helping professions* (4th ed.). Open University Press.

Holloway, E. (1995). *Clinical supervision: A systems approach.* Sage Publications.

Kagan, H., & Kagan, N. (1997). Interpersonal process recall: Influencing human interaction. In C. E. Watkins, Jr. (Ed.), *Handbook of psychotherapy supervision* (pp. 296–309). Wiley.

Reed, D. A. (2019). Internal Family Systems informed supervision: A grounded theory inquiry (Identifier ETD2019Reed). Doctoral Dissertation, *St. Mary's University Digital Commons Repository.* https://commons.stmarytx.edu/dissertations/27.

Schwartz, R. C. (1995). *Internal Family Systems therapy*. The Guilford Press.

Schwartz, R. C. (2013). The therapist–client relationship and the transformative power of Self. In M. Sweezy & E. Ziskind (Eds.), *Internal Family Systems therapy: New dimensions* (pp. 1–23). Routledge.

Schwartz, R. C., & Sweezy, M. (2020). *Internal Family Systems therapy* (2nd ed.). The Guilford Press.

3 Facilitating Flow

Developing a Framework for Integrating IFS and Supervision in Private Practice in the UK

Liz Martins

Introduction

My phone rings, and when I answer it is a therapist and supervisor, just off a Level 1 training, seeking supervision. She is excited and keen to put her learning into practice. I notice that I am leaning forward in response, wanting to support her in taking IFS to her clients and supervisees. She asks whether supervision based on the IFS model is any different to the supervision she is used to. I love her question and tell her so. I share that exploring this question has been an ongoing journey for me over recent years.

After training in IFS I integrated the model fully into my therapy practice with my clients. IFS is the map for my work, the lens that I look through, the pathway that I follow. However, in my supervision and consultation practice with individuals and groups, it was less straightforward. I supervise therapists with varying levels of training in and experience of IFS as well as therapists who have no familiarity with the model. My original training as a therapist was in psychosynthesis, while my supervision training was based on traditional therapy models, including psychodynamic and person-centred. As I became more experienced with IFS, I wondered how to integrate it more deeply into my supervision practice. I could talk *about* IFS with supervisees (and did so often), but was there something in *how* I worked? Was there something different in the goals, the focus, the process of IFS supervision?

I am fortunate to have experienced rich learning from working with experienced IFS supervisors/consultants and trainers, particularly Cece Skyes, Osnat Arbel, and Susan McConnell, and I have learned a great deal from observing Richard Schwartz in his consultancy work. I found Dan Read's PhD research on IFS-informed supervision useful (Reed, 2019) and attended his workshop at the IFS Conference in 2019. However, there is relatively little written about IFS and supervision, so the development of my supervision style has mostly come from reflective practicing and from experiencing IFS consultation. More recently, Emma Redfern and I began an ongoing conversation about IFS and supervision, exploring what our

DOI: 10.4324/9781003044864-3

practice involves when we are informed by and in the flow of IFS. Following this U-turning together, we developed a model for IFS supervision and now share this in workshops.

Integrating IFS into supervision is still a work in progress for me. However, over time, my practice has developed and deepened into something that to me feels like IFS. This chapter describes my journey and shows how I have applied the aspects that have become most central to my practice. At the end, I share a simple framework for IFS Supervision that emerged from my learning and forms part of the model developed with Emma Redfern (see Chapter 14).

In this chapter, I refer to *supervision* rather than consultation, as this is the term most commonly used in the UK regardless of the stage of training and development of the therapist. Similarly, I use the term *therapist* or *supervisee* rather than consultee.

Following the IFS Model: From "Doing Supervision" to "Being an IFS Supervisor"

I started my journey as a supervisor with my managers and supervising parts to the fore. They believed that supervision was about therapists coming with the stories of their clients and that after I had listened, I should offer wise suggestions for what they should do in their next session. I also had some caretaking parts that enquired about the therapist, maybe at times getting a little protective or indignant on their behalf. My intellectual parts were aware of parallel process, so occasionally I checked inside and, if it seemed relevant, I shared what I was noticing, for example, anxiety or fogginess. Then my intellectual parts and the thinking parts of the therapist might have a conversation about what that might mean. I also had parts that did not feel good enough as a supervisor, particularly with therapists more experienced than me, and sometimes these parts were present in the room to control my input, turning it up or down.

I am exaggerating, but not as much as I would like. Looking back, my system was parts-led much of the time and so was my supervision practice. I remember that in those days some of my parts even became a little impatient sometimes as we talked about how the therapist was at the beginning of the session, as this seemed a distraction to the main business of our meeting. My managers liked to make a list of the clients the therapist wanted to present and off we would go. I was definitely "doing supervision."

The IFS model provides us with "a clear, nonpathologizing, empowering, user-friendly map" (Schwartz, 2013, p. 22). The shift, the realization, that I have made over time is that this map is just as relevant to supervision as it is to therapy (and indeed to living life). It offers all that is needed, starting with the goals of IFS: restoring trust in Self-leadership, achieving balance and harmony, releasing parts from extreme roles, and bringing more Self-energy to the world. IFS could be a guide to my practice and process in supervision, and I could turn to the model when the flow of my work was stuck or uncertain. As I started to learn this, it changed my way of being a supervisor.

Quite early in my practice I was working with a supervisee, Jim, who had a client with a very complex inner system following childhood trauma. Over many years Jim sat with this client while the protectors blasted him with anger and criticism. Occasionally, Jim glimpsed an exile, desperate and alone, before the protectors stepped back in to take control. In our supervision sessions we discussed direct access, the 6 Fs, and how to negotiate with the protectors. Gradually, over time, we shifted. We started to slow down, to sit back. We spent gentle time attending to Jim's parts that found being with the client's protectors triggering. We softened into appreciation and compassion for the client's protectors that were working so hard. Together, we found ways to hold patience, trust, and hope. IFS supervision stopped being about IFS theory and became embodied and real. One day Jim came to supervision excited. He told me that for a few moments, he and his client had connected in a way that was completely new. He described it as being like a ray of light breaking through for a magical moment.

The client's protectors had stepped back in by the next session but, over time, more Self-energy became available and, eventually, some of the client's exiles were unburdened. For me, I was learning lessons about partnering with the IFS model in my supervision. If all participants in the supervisory system have a Self, then the wisdom is already in the system. My role was not to know or to be the expert about the client's system or the supervisee's practice, but rather to bring my expertise in IFS to maximize access to Self-energy. I could be a curious, kind partner in exploration, rather than an expert figuring it out (Schwartz & Sweezy, 2020). This was a radical shift for some of my supervisor parts. However, they stepped back, and I started to settle in my chair.

I was slowing down. At the beginning of group or individual sessions, I began to invite supervisees to spend a few moments inside, to connect to and hear from their parts about what needed our attention. A supervisee, Louise, arrived with some clients to discuss, but when she went inside, immediately an image came of a different client that she was due to see later that day. As we stayed with this, she discovered parts that were frightened of a critical part of her client. As she heard more, it turned out that they were confusing the client with a critical teacher in her past. Louise was able to unblend and update her frightened parts and felt positive about the session to come.

I was learning to offer more spaciousness and internal connection. My focus was shifting from the client to focusing as much on the therapist and their internal system. I noticed that I was using my IFS skills of working with the 6 Fs, using in-sight and direct access, just as I would in client sessions. Occasionally, we might not get to discussing clients at all and stay working with the therapist's system. As with my client work, I brought conscious intention to be collaborative and transparent as well as to contract for where we went, both at the outset of our work and in the moment. The difference, of course, was that this was not a therapy session, and I would hold in mind that our purpose always was to be in service of the supervisee's work with their current and future clients.

Another challenge for me was how to bring IFS into my supervision with therapists who were not IFS-informed and had no intention of training in IFS. I began to realize that IFS can be our modality as supervisors whatever the approach of the supervisee. With someone not trained in IFS, I use more implicit direct access, less going inside and reduced use of IFS terminology and parts language. However, the IFS lens is just as relevant to my work. I am explicit in my initial contracting that IFS is the frame of my understanding and that I "translate" into the language and modality of the supervisee as we work. Where there is interest, I offer the IFS perspective.

In these ways, as my supervision practice developed, I was coming more into partnership with the IFS model and trusting the Self-energy in the system. I was slowing down, offering more choice, more space, letting go of having to be the one who knows and shifting to a more collaborative way of working.

Taking a Systemic Perspective: Bringing Clarity and Calm

Fortunately, my training as a supervisor included a systems perspective that was based on the Seven-eyed Model of Supervision (Hawkins & Shohet, 2012). This model details seven lenses or systems for a supervisor to consider in their work. For me, IFS brought greater richness and depth and widened my perspective further, drawing attention to the interconnected web of systems of Self and parts. Attention can be scaled up to the organizational, cultural, or global contexts, and down to the Self and parts within a person's internal system, and then further down to the Self and parts of these parts (Schwartz, 2021). Beyond even these systems, IFS offers a perspective across time with attention to intergenerational legacy burdens and heirlooms (Sinko, 2017; Henriques & Shull, 2021), and wider to a sense of a realm beyond our understanding inhabited by unattached burdens and guides (Falconer, 2021).

In supervision, I was becoming more attuned to the internal system of each of the participants (client, therapist, supervisor) set within our external contexts of family, work, and other networks. I was also becoming more aware of the relational fields between these overlapping systems. I began to notice and address the polarizations and alliances, for example, drawing attention to where a therapist's manager was allied with the managers in a client's external family system trying to stop a firefighter drinking, or where parts of a therapist were allying with client parts, telling me about a "terrible husband" whilst ignoring the parts that were staying in the relationship.

Training in Intimacy From the Inside Out (IFIO) supported me to better track the dynamics between parts of a client and parts of a therapist (Herbine-Blank et al., 2016). For example, in one supervision session, a therapist and I tracked how, with a particular client, the supervisee's exile that did not feel good enough got triggered and activated one of her protectors that then withdrew her from the relationship. We noticed how this seemed to activate the client's exile that felt abandoned, and this then activated the client's critical/blaming protector. The therapist part that did not feel good enough then reacted to the criticism and so on.

Just noticing this dynamic helped the therapist to unblend and find more compassion and understanding for her client's system as well as for her own. She reported that next time her client's critical/blaming part let her know that therapy was not helping, rather than getting blended with the "not good enough" part, she was able to express appreciation to the client for sharing and offer validation to this part for what it was feeling. This led to the client being able to unblend from the blaming part and speak for another part's fear that she was not doing therapy "right." They went on to meet and unburden this part, who was eight years old and stuck in a scene in school.

In recent years, the impact of events happening in systems outside the supervision space has become far more obvious. For example, the cultural, societal, political, and global influences of the Black Lives Matter and #MeToo movements, the climate emergency, Brexit, and the COVID-19 pandemic all show up in supervision as our protectors and exiles (including mine) react. The fear, loss, and loneliness of the COVID-19 pandemic is triggering for young parts already holding these burdens and, in supervision, I am attentive to what is "the past" and what are "present time" reactions. I notice that IFS provides a map either way – the healing steps to unburdening the past or Self connecting to parts suffering in the present, which helps prevent burdens being developed and taken forward.

Importantly, these global events heightened my awareness of some of the cultural and legacy burdens that impact on supervision, including racism and patriarchy. The work of Kate Lingren and Percy Ballard helps me to acknowledge and understand the implicit bias held within my own system and to assume its presence in my supervisees also, and it offers ways to be with parts that are holding these burdens (see Kate Lingren's Chapter 9). This is ongoing personal work for me within a larger context where Richard Schwartz offers us hope that once a critical mass of collective Self is reached then large-scale healing will happen (Schwartz, 2021).

Thus, over time, I was becoming more aware that I operate within a multiplicity of systems and times, a wider interconnected field of Self and parts, as well as burdens of many kinds and at all levels. The systemic frame of IFS brings a sense of a bigger picture that is helpful and hopeful. It gives more of a long-term view to help supervisees look back to notice progress made and to look forward with a vision of healing to come over time. It helps me to validate and normalize, to see the size and place of what we are with, and therefore I am more able to let go and just be with. The 8 Facets Model developed with Emma Redfern (see Chapter 14) helps me to be more flexible, to zoom in and out, offering a systemic map with options of where to focus and supervision questions that I might ask.

This wider perspective brings calm and clarity to my system, which benefits my supervisees in turn. Rather than supervision narrowly focusing on the therapist as we consider their work with a particular client, for me it is now more like time spent together in a vast field of Self-energy and parts "beyond ideas of wrongdoing and rightdoing" (Rumi, 2004, p. 36). I also know in my bones that compassion and acceptance are contagious and can seep through the cracks into all levels of all systems (Schwartz, 2013), and I am able to add my contribution through my supervision practice.

Favoring Stuckness: Moving from Content to Process

As in my early client work, my early supervision sessions generally started with me listening to a story. Supervisees told me about a client, their history and presenting issues, and their work with the client. Sometimes therapists spoke for or from parts that were responding to the client. I became curious about who in the therapist's system was choosing to present this particular client and why. Sometimes supervisees brought their successes to share and celebrate. However, mostly the client featured because the work was complex and challenging, or it impacted on them, or they were stuck in some way.

As I continued to deepen into integrating IFS into my supervision practice, I became less interested in the story and more focused on listening for the parts involved, including who was narrating. Inspired by the work of Cece Sykes, who uses an inverted triangle to represent an inner system (Sykes, 2017), I began to map the parts that I was hearing, using three triangles – one for the client, one for the therapist, and one for my system, with lines coming in to represent external influences, including legacy burdens. I often share these maps with supervisees.

Mostly, I was learning to listen for if (or where) the work was stuck. My intention was to get a sense of the territory and then shift attention to where the healing pathway was blocked or needed support. With some presentations, this would be clear. The therapist might even name it. For example, Sarah, a supervisee, told me, "I just can't find a way in. She just turns up and talks about anything and everything, and I can't get past it." Other times, the supervisee and I explored how the work was flowing and then agreed our focus for supervision, in a similar way to identifying what IFS therapy calls a *target part* (Schwartz & Sweezy, 2020). Sometimes I just learned to wait patiently and track closely, trusting that what needed attention would emerge.

"When we encounter a problem in therapy, it means that a part is probably interfering – but we don't know whose part it is: the client's or ours" (Schwartz & Sweezy, 2020, p. 89). Over time, I noticed some common patterns within and between the client and supervisee systems. For example, Sarah (mentioned earlier) was frustrated that her client just talked and talked. Other therapists told me about "endless protectors" or asked me about how to get this or that one to step back. Often, with some exploration, we would find a stand-off between the helping or "doing IFS" parts of the therapist, which wanted the client's protector(s) to move out of the way, and the protector(s) of the client, which sensed the therapist's intention for change. The client's protectors were digging in and not going anywhere anytime soon. When Sarah realized that the talking came from a protector, she got interested in and even impressed by its hard work of creating wall-to-wall conversation as a protective tactic. As Sarah softened and her frustrated parts relaxed back, she had more curiosity and, within a few sessions, sensing her Self-energy, the client's talking part had agreed to give more space.

I came to notice how the work stalled when therapist parts held a story of inadequacy. This was particularly evident in my supervision for an agency offering a counseling service to people with significant childhood trauma, which was often provided by inexperienced or student therapists. I found this challenging as a supervisor, more so as my supervisees were not IFS-informed. When their work was stuck, we would notice and stay with this, often meeting the parts that felt overwhelmed, lost, and not skilled enough. I would welcome these parts, validating and normalizing their fears. As they were given time and space, sometimes to cry, the parts would start to settle, with more calm becoming available in the system.

I would encourage these novice therapists to let go of "helping" and to focus on finding their curiosity and compassion, suggesting that it could be immensely powerful for their clients to experience this when perhaps it had not been offered before. Often this would seem to release something in the dynamic between the therapist and their client, and the work would deepen. Working in this agency helped me develop more ways to bring IFS to my supervision practice without mentioning IFS or using the language of parts. I realized that the process in supervision of noticing and focusing on the blocks to progression in the work was the same as unblending and accessing Self-energy.

Sometimes the flow was stalled for different reasons. John, an experienced therapist new to IFS, wanted to discuss that his work "never seems to get to unburdening." With the permission of a client, he brought a recording of his work for us to watch in supervision. We observed that, as the client's protector started to hint at the exile underneath – a toddler crying in a cot – a part of John started to ask about the client's relationship with his partner. The client enthusiastically engaged with that, the focus veered away, and they did not return to the exile. Watching the video, John was mystified about why he had changed the subject in the way he had, but when he checked inside, he found a part that believed that the toddler's distress would have been too much and would have got out of control. This helped me get interested in the subtle ways that therapists' protectors sometimes form implicit alliances with clients' protectors to avoid the pain held by the client's exiles.

In my supervision practice, therefore, I was learning to give priority to where the work was stuck and to listen deeply for the parts involved, rather than being distracted by the details of the history or presentation. Sometimes this required slowing down and unblending from my impatient parts, which became easier as I did my own work in therapy and found greater calm and more trust within my own system.

Freeing Up Self-Energy: Working with Parts

According to Schwartz (2013, see pp. 21–22), the quality of presence brings the capacity to open to and enhance connection with the larger, transcendent Self and allows the work to flow, with space for insight and solutions to emerge. He states that, "It is not possible to do therapy without having parts taking over at times," and what is needed is an "exquisitely sensitive parts detector" (Schwartz, 2013, p. 16). My supervision practice became more focused on parts detecting.

Of course, I needed to start with my own system. I brought learning from IFS, somatic IFS, and IFIO (Intimacy from the Inside Out) trainings into my supervision practice as I found ways to U-turn. I would ask myself, "How do I feel toward … ?" and check my thoughts, emotions, impulses, body, breathing, and my heart. This all helped me become familiar with my parts that want to give advice; to teach; to caretake supervisees and/or their clients; to be liked, needed, and valued.

I learned to be especially watchful for a part that thinks it knows, that leans forward, gets a little "up" with excitement and wants to share its insight with the supervisee into what is going on with the client's system. Sometimes it has something useful to contribute. However, I seek to be Self-led in how this part's contribution might be brought into the supervision space, taking a moment to breathe, to reconnect my back with my chair, to check inside, and then to ask the supervisee if hearing from this part would be welcome.

Sometimes I notice a part that has been triggered by a connection with my personal history or parts that hold assumptions and biases absorbed from my cultural and historical context, and these become trailheads for me. Often my parts bring helpful information, illuminating something that is taking place in the supervisory relationship or between therapist and client, commonly known as parallel process (Hawkins & Shohet, 2012). Over time I have learned to respect and trust my parts much more and now deeply value how they help me in my work. For example, a supervisee tells me about a session with her client, and when I name that my chest is tight and it is hard to breathe, it turns out that this accurately reflects her experience of the therapy session, with little space and a lack of movement in the work.

I discovered that I need to be attentive, particularly initially, to any supervisee parts that are triggered by the supervision process itself, to make space for Self-leadership. For example, a supervisee, Clara, had a part that felt uncomfortable in supervision because it learned many years ago at school that it was unsafe to show her work. We needed to attend to this part before it would give her enough space to freely discuss her work with me. The part now sits beside her in our sessions.

Ever more aware of my White privilege and implicit bias, when working with supervisees who are Black or people of color I became more sensitive to parts in the room holding personal, cultural, or legacy burdens with beliefs and expectations connected to racism and power. As with other issues of difference, such as gender and sexual orientation, I found ways to name this with my supervisees, so that our differences can be acknowledged and parts spoken for. I encourage supervisees to do the same with their clients.

I noticed that many therapists have parts that are harshly critical of their work. These parts tell them that if their client had a different, more competent therapist, they would be healed by now. I noticed how the young parts that believe this and hold the shame of not being skilled enough can find supervision a difficult and exposing experience. This may be exacerbated if these parts have experienced a female parent or teacher who has been critical or dismissive, and they expect that of me.

I learned to anticipate that these therapist parts would be around somewhere and look out for them or even gently invite the therapist to speak for them. I learned to slow down, to put aside the clients and really attend with gentleness and care to these parts of my supervisees, to give space and acceptance, to help them to notice and build trust in the therapist's Self. I felt a lot of tenderness for these parts given that I have my own plentiful experience of shaming and shamed parts in my system too and know how hard this can make the experience of supervision.

Attending to these parts makes more room to notice the parts of the therapist that come up in response to their work with clients. Inviting a U-turn, we would discover parts connected to the therapist's personal history, triggered by an association with an emotion, topic, or scene. For example, with one supervisee, Maria, we started to notice a blocking part. This part would filter out information about her clients' relationships with their fathers as if this was unimportant. It was as if it was forbidden territory for this part, leaving the therapist with a blind spot. As we noticed this, it became a trailhead and, in her therapy, she worked with the protector and then with the exile that held enormous grief about the absence of her own father, who left the family home when she was four.

Another supervisee discovered that a protector was not allowing her to say "No" to prospective clients. It turned out that this protector thought that she was nine and was trying to prevent a repeat of the child being bullied and rejected at school. Once the part was updated and noticed Self, it was willing to trust the therapist to manage her client appointments. Boundaries (or the lack of them), including issues around frequency of sessions, overrunning, not charging for late cancellations, and contact between sessions, form a common theme. I learned to get curious with the therapist about who is making these decisions and whether they are Self- or parts-led decisions.

For example, when a supervisee, Frances, told me she planned to increase the number of sessions per week with a client, she agreed to explore this more with me. It turned out that a young part of Frances was fearful of a demanding protector part of the client, who was insistent that more sessions were needed. With a history of conflict in her own family, Frances's part wanted to avoid the anticipated anger in response to a "No." After unblending from the fearful part in supervision, Frances decided not to go ahead with increasing the sessions and, instead, in her next session with the client, worked with the client's insistent, demanding part. This led to the client meeting, with the permission of the protector, an exile desperate for connection. Frances facilitated the client's Self-to-exile relationship in the session and the client committed to maintaining that connection between sessions. This satisfied the client's parts and the additional therapy sessions were no longer sought.

Another common theme is the presence of Self-like parts of therapists – parts that hold many qualities of Self but have more of an agenda, for example, to help, fix, or rescue. The work of Osnat Arbel (2021) helped me to discern when there was some energy of action or doing that hinted at a Self-like part taking charge of a therapist's work. Often these are young caretaking parts. I also commonly meet therapist parts that have trained for many years, read numerous books about therapy, and step in to do the work (much like my supervisee parts mentioned earlier). Other protectors worry about not being effective or not being liked by their clients. As an IFS supervisor, I learned to listen out for exile beliefs, for example, *I always get it wrong, I'm not enough, I will be rejected*.

Where a supervisee's part is playing a significant role in the therapeutic process, I see my role as helping the supervisee notice its presence, notice the trailhead. Then there are choices to be made about how far to progress along the healing pathway from just noticing the part, to unblending and building the Self-to-protector relationship, to working with an exile through to unburdening. On the one hand, I know that the more therapist Self-energy is available, the more this will help the client. On the other hand, this is supervision, not a therapy session, and there are strong arguments (including from regulatory organizations) that boundaries between the two are best kept clear and well maintained.

As I deepened into my supervision practice, I found my own way with this. I am clear that my primary purpose is the benefit of the therapist's clients, and I discuss the supervision/therapy boundary at initial contract and then contract on an ongoing basis with the supervisee. I check in the moment where we are and where we might go, particularly if we are heading deeper into the therapist's own system and history. I might offer the option to go deeper but hold this more lightly than I would in a therapy session with a client, where there is more of an intention for healing. Factors influencing the depth to which we work include whether the supervisee is in therapy, whether the setting is individual or group, the time available, and the impact of the part on the therapist's work.

As my practice developed, most supervision sessions involved noticing therapist parts, frequently involved working with protectors to unblend, perhaps building the Self-to-part relationship and updating the part about the client's Self. Occasionally, we would meet and work with exiles; more rarely, a supervision session featured the unburdening of an exile.

Fostering Fluency in IFS: Building Understanding and Skills

As well as slowing down, prioritizing stuckness, and working with parts, as I deepened into integrating IFS into my supervision offering, I also focused on supporting each supervisee to develop their own practice. For many, this was specifically about learning IFS, which is why they were working with me. My image for this was of helping supervisees to learn how to ski – moving and adapting to the conditions, being in their bodies rather than their minds, feeling free and fluent as they traverse the IFS healing pathway.

My parts that love to teach enjoy this aspect of supervision. Although there might often be a discussion about some aspect of IFS, for example, how to work with legacy unburdening or ways to unblend, I also find that supervisees find it helpful when I "translate into IFS" what I hear them say. So, I might listen and then repeat in parts language. I might reflect on how their work fitted with the protocol, for example, "It sounds like you were doing some beautiful work there building the Self-to-part relationship." Sometimes, watching a video of their work or doing a *real-play* (where the supervisee or I takes on the role of their client with the other as the therapist) gives me an opportunity to teach. I also watch for the C qualities in their practice and name the courage, the compassion, the moments of connection that I observe.

Over time, I have become more conscious of teaching IFS by trying to model it and "walk the talk" myself. For example, I make visible that I am taking a moment to unblend, speak for my parts, and apologize for them where necessary. With agreement, I try to offer experience of IFS in practice, inviting supervisees to go inside and come into relationship with their parts and hear from them.

As I gained experience as an IFS supervisor, I became familiar with and able to anticipate some of the places where inexperienced IFS therapists might struggle. For example, some find it hard to facilitate their clients moving from telling their story to bringing their attention inside, or they give insufficient attention to building Self-to-part relationships. Some beginning IFS therapists lack confidence in working with and unburdening exiles. I have become used to gently reminding less experienced IFS therapists that they could ask the client, rather than asking me.

To return to the skiing metaphor, sometimes the snow is bumpy – supervisees lose their balance or their confidence, even falling occasionally. I gently encourage persistence; offer hope, trust, and confidence; and support them in picking themselves up and going round again to keep going. One supervisee regularly started our sessions with "I just can't do this IFS thing." However, she persisted, and eventually she started to find more ease, more fluency, more enjoyment in her IFS work. Sometimes I too would hit a bump in my practice and fall over, perhaps my parts misunderstanding or inadvertently shaming, and I would apologize and seek repair.

With supervisees not trained in IFS, my focus, my map, is similar, but without IFS teaching or language. I encourage supervisees to slow down, to befriend the protection in the system, to offer and invite hope and curiosity, and to invite clients to notice in the moment what happens to their thoughts, body, emotions. We might talk about how they can support their clients to find compassion so that they can "sit with their sadness" or "be with the child inside who that happened to." I have parts that find it frustrating sometimes to work in a different language and to be so aware of the potential for healing that IFS could bring to their clients.

In these ways, I sought to free confidence and clarity in my supervisees, and I noticed that when these qualities were more abundant, the supervisees had more compassion available for and toward their clients. In turn, this brought more connection. I was also learning to ski in my supervision practice, to feel the joyfulness of navigating the twists and turns, with my parts finding more confidence to trust me and allow me to be in the flow of my work.

Firing Up Creativity: Going Beyond Talking

As I gained confidence, I started to bring in more lightness, more playfulness. It was natural for me, as my parts relaxed, to invite in more fun and, in turn, this seemed to enable some of the parts of my supervisees that hold burdened beliefs to relax also, giving us more space for connection. I started to experiment with inviting supervisees to join me in working in other ways than our usual pattern of talking about. What might we find out if we came at it differently?

For example, when a supervisee's parts are reacting to a client, I occasionally use a *firedrill*, which is a technique taught in IFS training. This is a guided meditation where the client is evoked using imagination, with them doing or saying whatever it is that triggers the therapist. The therapist is then guided through a U-turn to meet their reactive protector(s) and then possibly to meet the exile that they are protecting. I also sometimes use objects, images, or drawings to externalize parts and encourage their expression. In a group setting, participants can embody parts of the client or the supervisee, and the global pandemic has drawn my attention to the creative opportunities of working outside in nature.

My parts trained in Sensorimotor Psychotherapy love to work with embodiment and movement, and I began to experiment with working with my supervisees in this way. For example, we might explore boundaries with a string laid on the floor or study endings through letting go of an object and noticing what parts come up. Where parts show up in gestures and impulses, we slow down and explore the movement, for example, to push or turn away, to reach out or step toward. When we started working together, one therapist introduced her clients to me through embodying each of them without words. This helped us get a sense of their Self and parts.

I might invite a real-play where I play the therapist and my supervisee takes on the role of their client. This often brings surprising insights. For example, a therapist who had only experienced her client's pleasing, compliant parts "discovered" that the client had a gatekeeping protector that "totally doesn't trust me." Training in somatic IFS gave me other ideas that I work with, for example, about listening in different ways, from the front or back of the body, or with "radical resonance" (McConnell, 2020). For example, with one therapist we worked with her listening deeply inside to notice how her body responded as I repeated back to her what she had been telling me about her client, and she became aware of a part that wanted to shrink away.

As I started to work more with people who were seeking to be certified in IFS, I became alive to the potential of observing videos of the work of supervisees. Often, it is illuminating to discover the gap between how therapists present their work and how it actually is in practice. These supervision sessions, in which we watch and discuss practice, feel rich and useful to supervisees, and they are more effective than hearing second hand about their work with clients.

In these ways, I have embraced bringing something more creative into supervision, to make it more engaging (for me, as well as for supervisees), and to give parts other ways to be seen and heard. I hope that in turn this encourages supervisees to bring playfulness and creativity into their work also.

Drawing It All Together: A Framework for Supervision

This, then, is an account of my journey and learning to integrate IFS into my work as a supervisor. Over time I have learned to follow the IFS model and use it to guide my supervision, coming into partnership with Self, with the model, and with the supervisee. With greater awareness of the systems involved, I have gained perspective and turn toward places where the flow of the work is blocked. Attending to the parts involved in these places has become my focus, whether they are the parts of the client or of the therapist, knowing from IFS that if more Self-energy can be accessed, then the therapeutic work can better flow toward the healing that the client desires and deserves.

As my practice shifted toward freeing up Self-energy, I embraced the practice of enabling the therapist to become ever more proficient with IFS. I became more skilled, more persistent, perhaps more kind, in how I help supervisees learn and deepen their understanding and skills. Finally, on my journey I got more creative and playful in how I work.

In my conversations with Emma Redfern, this learning has surfaced into a simple framework:

The Fs and Ps of IFS Supervision:

> FOLLOW the model – Partnership
> FRAME systemically – Perspective
> FAVOR stuckness – Patience
> FREE UP Self-energy – Presence
> FOSTER fluency – Persistence
> FIRE UP creativity – Playfulness

(© 2020 Liz Martins and Emma E. Redfern)

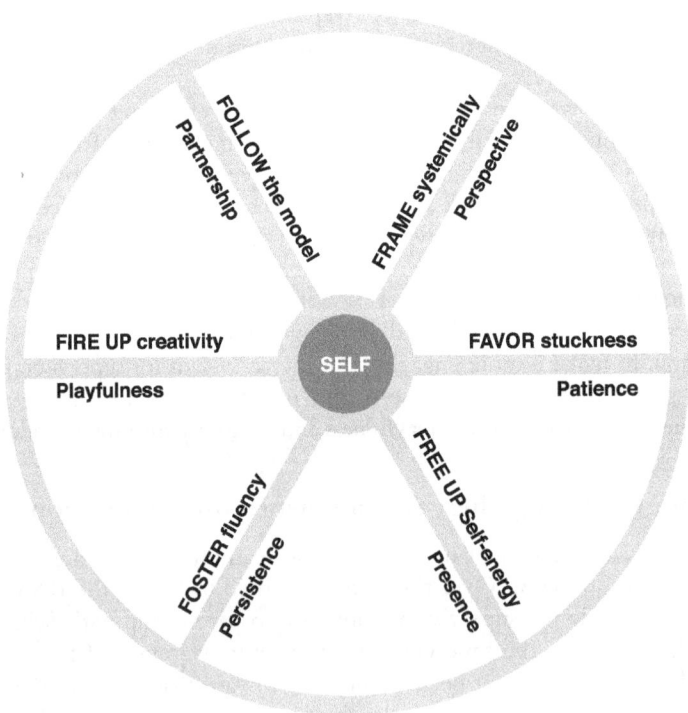

Figure 3.1 The Fs and Ps of IFS Supervision

The Fs in the framework form an extension to, and are inspired by, the 6 Fs that we know from IFS. Each F suggests a direction or focus, and they are paired with the qualities of Self-led therapists, as set out by Schwartz and known as the 5 Ps with the addition of an extra P – Partnership. In practice the pairs are not sequential and are interconnected. This framework is now supporting me in my supervision practice with individuals and groups. I use it to steer by, for example, checking the P qualities that are present and moving towards whichever F seems to be needed (see Figure 3.1).

Schwartz says that IFS is essentially a map to the sacred place that involves the "ineffable touching of spirits" (Schwartz, 2013, p. 22). There was little sacred about my supervision practice when I began, but now I hope that, as well as supportive challenge, it holds light, clarity, hope, kindness, welcome, and even love. Through IFS I have been given "clear-cut ways to ensure that the relationship is filled with Self-energy" (Schwartz, 2013, p. 22). If this is so with supervision, then I trust there will be more Self-energy available for the therapists' clients in turn and that this will bring them healing. As I responded on the phone to the question of a newly-trained IFS therapist, I was able to tell her, "Yes, IFS has changed the way that I offer supervision, and I am deeply grateful for that."

References

Arbel, O. (2021). The Self-led therapist [MOOC]. *LifeArchitect*. https://lifearchitect.com/self-led-ifs-therapist.

Falconer, R. (2021). The further reaches of IFS: Unattached burdens and guides [MOOC]. *LifeArchitect*.

Hawkins, P., & Shohet, R. (2012). *Supervision in the helping professions* (4th ed.). Open University Press.

Henriques, A., & Shull, T. (2021, January 3). IFS Talks: Legacy burdens and heirlooms: A talk with Osnat Arbel [Audio podcast episode]. *Apple Podcasts*. https://podcasts.apple.com/gb/podcast/legacy-burdens-and-heirlooms-a-talk-with-osnat-arbel/id1481000501?i=1000504208855

Herbine-Blank, T., Kerpelman, D. M., & Sweezy, M. (2016). *Intimacy from the inside out: Courage and compassion in couple therapy*. Routledge.

McConnell, S. (2020). *Somatic Internal Family Systems therapy*. North Atlantic Books.

Reed, D. A. (2019). Internal Family Systems informed supervision: A grounded theory inquiry (Identifier ETD2019Reed). Doctoral Dissertation, *St. Mary's University Digital Commons Repository*. https://commons.stmarytx.edu/dissertations/27.

Rumi (2004). *Selected Poems*. Translated by Coleman Barks. Penguin Classics.

Schwartz, R. C. (2013). The therapist–client relationship and the transformative power of Self. In M. Sweezy & E. L. Ziskind (Eds.), *Internal Family Systems therapy: New dimensions* (pp. 1–23). Routledge.

Schwartz, R. C. (2021, February 26–28). Heirloom Summit 2021: Transforming legacy burdens to legacy gifts [online event].

Schwartz, R. C., & Sweezy, M. (2020). *Internal Family Systems therapy* (2nd ed.). The Guilford Press.

Sinko, A. L. (2017). Legacy burdens. In M. Sweezy & E. L. Ziskind (Eds.), *Innovations and elaborations in Internal Family Systems therapy* (pp. 164–178). Routledge.

Sykes, C. (2017). An IFS lens on addiction: Compassion for extreme parts. In M. Sweezy & E. L. Ziskind (Eds.), *Innovations and elaborations in Internal Family Systems therapy* (pp. 29–48). Routledge.

4 Parts Detecting Across Multiple Systems

The Application of IFS in Consultation to Therapists of Children and Adolescents

Pamela K. Krause

This chapter explains how to supervise child therapists from the perspective of Internal Family Systems therapy (IFS).[1] First and foremost, the IFS consultant makes the journey to Self-leadership by delving into their own internal system. From there, the job of the IFS consultant is to help consulting therapists delve into three internal systems of parts – their own, the child's, and the parents' – with special attention to polarizations and alliances within and between all of these systems. Along the way, I offer examples of some of my parts activating along with case examples from consultations, which are an amalgam and do not represent any individual therapist or client. For the purposes of this chapter, the word *child* describes any minor, a child, or an adolescent, while the word *parent* describes the child's caretakers.

But before going into all that, I'll say a few words about myself. I learned to love working with children and adolescents during field placements in graduate school. A few years later, in 1998, I started a private practice and began to train in IFS therapy. At the time, trainings did not offer specific guidance for this population and few people used the IFS model with young people. As a result, I developed my own way of applying IFS with kids and began teaching it. By 2005, I was a lead trainer for the IFS Institute, teaching the first two levels of training. At the same time, I developed a program for child therapists and contributed chapters on the topic to two different textbooks: "IFS with Children and Adolescents" (Krause, 2013) and "EMDR Therapy and the Use of Internal Family Systems Strategies With Children" with Ana Gomez (Gomez & Krause, 2013). Finally, I've offered individual and group consultation on child therapy for the last 12 years. Since I apply IFS across the board, I am client-led as I practice therapy and therapist-led when I consult. I keep the child's needs front and center.

IFS child therapy includes a complex relational web and, in my experience, it is very effective with children. In addition to the child, we see the child's parents, sometimes other members of the extended family, and sometimes community members who are involved with the child. This means we will interact with adults who are at various levels of being blended with vigilant protectors and whose personal agendas often conflict.

DOI: 10.4324/9781003044864-4

While our job is to be Self-led, people who are blended with extreme protectors can be a big challenge to attaining and maintaining Self-leadership. The more complex the relational web, the greater the potential for one or more of the people involved to evoke our protective parts. Therefore, the primary goal of consultation is to help therapists get clear about their own parts: which ones are active, what happened to activate them, and are they willing to unblend and allow the therapist's Self to take the lead?

In a process that is parallel to therapy, IFS consultation involves helping parts unblend and accessing the Self. The IFS consultant starts by helping their own activated parts unblend so they can be curious about the consulting therapist's blended parts. Once the consulting therapist's parts are willing to unblend, consultant and therapist move on together to notice and be curious about the child client's parts and the child's parents' parts. In this way, the consultant tracks four systems separately and in relation to each other. This is the complexity of child therapy consultation.

IFS Consultation

Let's look at IFS-based consultation along a continuum. The therapist chooses where to focus on this continuum during consultation sessions. At one end, consultation can focus on any parts of the consultant who get activated while listening to the therapist. One step in on this continuum, consultation can focus solely on the parts of the therapist who get activated by the child client or the parents. For example, if the therapist is afraid of a parent's anger, consultation would focus on helping the therapist track their fear back to the fearful part so they can unburden it (in consultation or on their own) and be Self-led with the angry parent. Another step in, the consultation could examine how the therapist's inner system interacts with the child's external systems, or how the inner systems of the parents and child interact, weaving in technical and theoretical aspects of IFS as needed. At the other end of the continuum, consultation focuses purely on the technical and theoretical aspects of IFS. In the example above, for instance, the therapist might have questions about how to use implicit or explicit direct access with the angry parent. Over time, most therapists choose to mix it up, spending one session discussing theory, the next on their own reactivity, and the next combining theory with internal inquiry into their parts. As with any interaction involving the IFS model, the person seeking help directs the session.

Self-Leadership as a Tool for Consultation

The Self-led internal system functions well because the Self and parts have mutual respect. The Self leads and parts give their input. No one is expendable, everyone is necessary, and neither parts nor Self is better or worse than the other. They are different and essential for our functioning.

Like many people, I experience the Self as the spiritual aspect of being and parts as the human, corporeal aspect of being. With Self-leadership we feel our parts and know them well, even when they are activated. They communicate with us constantly. Our Self is a resource for our parts and vice versa. When consulting, I have the opportunity to practice this way of being. I listen to my parts and learn from them, and they do the same. Their views and reactivity inform my consultations in crucial ways. For example, if my parts react to something the therapist says, it's likely that at least one other system (the child's, parents', or therapist's) has parts who are reacting in the same way. For this reason, I am transparent in consultation about what my parts feel and say.

Multiple Systems

The IFS consultant interacts, directly and indirectly, with multiple systems of parts and needs to focus on how these systems interface with and impact each other. They can include the consultant, therapist, child, parents, siblings, other family members, teachers, coaches, and more. I am focusing on four primary systems as a way of illustrating how systems interact with and impact each other. The possible combinations of these four interrelated systems include, but are not limited to:

> Parent/child
> Therapist/child
> Therapist/parents
> Therapist/parent and child
> Therapist/consultant

See Figure 4.1, where each system is represented by a circle.

Let's look at some possible polarizations and alignments. Each system interacts with other systems and contains its own polarizations and alignments. I'll take myself as an example. Over years of exploring, I've found a number of parts who routinely get activated when I consult. Although these can be embarrassing to acknowledge, they are common protectors in both therapists and consultants. My intellectual part often stands out first. This one wants to get all the details of the story so I can explain the theory of IFS to the consultee and teach them how to do it right. Following the intellectual part, I have one who judges the parents for their supposed bad parenting. This one polarizes with the parents and can feel anything from mild agitation to rage about what the parents are or are not doing. Then, a part who wants to be helpful to the therapist is also almost always present. It can be eager and talkative, offering many suggestions and ideas. If it senses the therapist's protectors are activated, especially if the therapist is feeling ashamed of something they've done, it can also be overly reassuring.

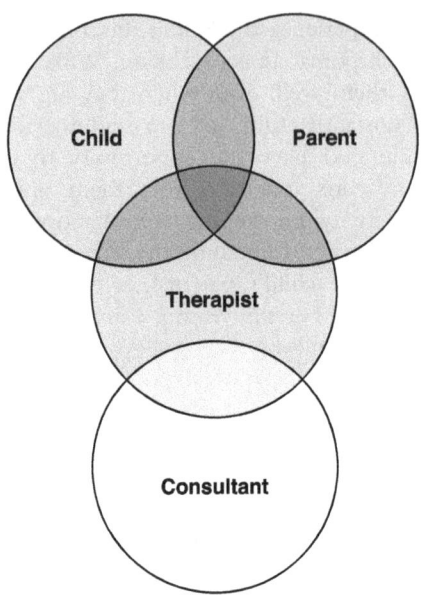

Figure 4.1 The Four Primary Systems

In the extreme, this reassuring part goes beyond eagerness to anxiety and urgency. A caring part who can masquerade as my Self generally shows up wanting to help and protect the child. This part can also pop up in cases where there are two parents because it believes one parent needs to be protected from the other. One part I find embarrassing gets frustrated with the therapist if they can't understand or implement my suggestions. But the part I'm most embarrassed about believes I'm a better IFS therapist than most and tells me I can do amazing work with this child.

Underneath these protectors I'm aware of some younger, more vulnerable parts. One feels unimportant and believes no one ever listens. This part emerges as an empty feeling in my throat and at the top part of my heart. Another vulnerable, empathic part resonates with all the pain in the world. This one is intuitive, and I experience it as an ache in my heart. Another can feel disconnected and unlovable. I experience it as a hollowness in my gut. And, finally, I have a part who can feel helpless and powerless. This list is not exhaustive. I'm just mentioning the ones who activate most often during consultation.

As you may realize from reading the passage above, I believe Self-leadership is a continuum running from full blending with no access to the Self to complete unblending with full access to the Self. The journey to Self-leadership, in my view, is lifelong. As an IFS consultant, I seek to be "Self-led enough", which means my parts are unblended enough that I experience my Self in relationship with them. I know it's possible, even probable, for external circumstances to activate my parts. Knowing they can, and sometimes will, knock me out of Self-leadership helps me accept the inevitable with enough grace to help them unblend more quickly. If I have difficulty returning to Self-leadership, I seek support from an IFS colleague or consultant.

Philip

Philip, a six-year-old boy, had been in therapy for six months. His biological mother brought him to therapy because of angry outbursts and aggressive behavior at home and in school. His parents were divorced, and he lived with his mother and a full brother, who was 18 months younger. Before divorcing, Philip's parents frequently fought. The father had been physically aggressive with the mother (i.e., grabbing, pushing her), but had never hit or punched her. Both parents had been verbally rageful. Around the age of two, Philip had begun to be aggressive with his mother, hitting and pushing her, calling her names, refusing to comply with her requests, and throwing things at her. Both parents had managed this aggression with aggression of their own. Although they didn't hit him, they got angry, yelled, grabbed him, and made him sit alone in a chair in another room. On the plus side, because they lived in a small house in a rural community with a temperate climate, Philip had been able to spend much of his time outside. His mother had worked from home most days, and her job had not been demanding.

After the divorce, Phillip's aggression did not increase in intensity or frequency, however he did show signs of anxiety, including having difficulty sleeping and biting his fingernails. He saw his father on weekends, and the therapist reported their relationship had been "good." Then his mother received a good job offer and moved the kids to a large, metropolitan city about a day's drive from the small rural community where they had been living and where their father still lived. After the move to the city, Philip's life changed drastically. He could not see his father for months at a time; his mother's job required her to work long hours, so she was only available for an hour in the morning and about three hours at the end of the day. The rest of the time he was at school, where he had recently begun kindergarten and after-school care. Their new apartment was "cramped" so he now shared a room with his brother. And, since they were in a large city, he now had little opportunity to play outside. Additionally, his mother began a relationship with a man who the therapist described as a "benign influence" in Philip's life, while also reporting that the man spent a great deal of time at their apartment, where he smoked pot, watched TV, and rarely interacted with the boys. As a result, Philip's behavior began to deteriorate. He became more aggressive with his mother and started being aggressive with his brother. He also began to have angry outbursts at school and aftercare. As his anxiety increased, he developed constant stomachaches and night terrors. The mother sought therapy at the school's insistence.

As the consultee presented this case, I tracked my parts' reactions and noticed the following parts. First, I was aware of a part who wanted more information. It felt urgent and excited and craved the details of the story so I could help. As I heard more of the story, my parts focused more on what happened to Philip, and I became aware of a caretaker who wanted to protect him and felt grief for everything that Philip had lost. Then I was aware of parts who felt hopeless and powerless, and I thought that was how Philip was feeling too.

Next, my focus shifted to the mother, and I noticed parts who were judging her for putting her needs over her children's needs. Not only did she take a new job and move her children away from their father, but she also got involved with another man quickly after the move. To top it off, the new guy was a "pot head." Finally, I noticed a part who was afraid of what could happen to Philip if someone didn't succeed in helping him to heal soon. I was concerned about his rage hurting him, his brother, his mother, and others, emotionally and physically.

As I listened to and acknowledged my parts' reactions, they unblended, and I became more Self-led. "Tell me where you're struggling and what would be helpful," I said to the consultee.

"I like Philip a lot," she replied, "He's a bright, funny little boy who just seems to need someone to pay attention to him. He hasn't gotten angry with me, but I have seen it because he's gotten angry with his mother in my waiting room."

Since this response did not answer my question, I asked again. "He hasn't gotten angry at you yet. So, where are you struggling with him or his mother?"

"I have a hard time with the mom. She's a nice woman, but I'm not sure she has much interest in Philip's therapy. Since she lets the boyfriend bring Philip most of the time, I hardly ever see her. I think that's not good for Philip. I don't think I can help him unless I can get his mom on board. I've tried a bunch of times to schedule something with mom, but she either doesn't respond or cancels."

"So, it sounds like we need to start with what's happening for you around the mom."

"Yes."

"Shall we start with your parts' reactions or with something like tracking parts of the mother, or how you two might be polarized or aligned?"

Just as an IFS therapist allows the client to choose where to begin, an IFS consultant does the same. This question invites the therapist to determine the framework for the consultation: internal inquiry, external systems, or interrelated systems. This therapist decided to start by exploring their own parts. "Are you aware of what gets triggered in you?" I asked.

"No, I'm not sure what's happening in me," they replied.

"Okay, let's try this. Remember a time when Mom didn't respond to your invitation to meet or canceled, and then let yourself *be* back there, at that moment. What do you notice?"

"That's so helpful! When I see her in front of me, I feel frustrated. Maybe even angry."

"Okay, anger comes first. Then what?"

"I think, I've told her this isn't going to work unless she's part of it. I've told her I can't help Philip without her support. But she seems to want me to fix him."

"Anything else?"

"Wow! I am angry with her. Not only does she fail to come in, but she has the nerve to be upset with me because Philip is still aggressive at home and school. She tells me that the school wants her to find a therapist who does CBT because Philip's behavior is still so bad."

"And what comes up when you hear that?"

"I've tried a million times to explain IFS to her. But she just can't – or won't – get it. I want to help Philip so much, but I feel helpless. And I'm so irritated I almost want to tell her to go ahead and take him somewhere else. But then I'm worried for Philip. I know CBT won't help him the way IFS could."

As the therapist talks, I hear many of the feelings and concerns that came up in me, including frustration, wanting to explain IFS to the mom, concern for Philip, and hopelessness.

"I hear a number of places where you could get curious," I said. "Where would you like to start?"

"All I can think is how concerned I am for Philip."

Since children usually live in a wounding environment with people who wound them, and therapy with children often needs to focus on present trauma as much as past trauma, child therapy often activates parts in the therapist and the consultant who love and want to protect the child. But caring, loving parts who want to fix things and hold people responsible are not the same as the Self. Many therapists find it challenging to distinguish between their Self-energy and their caring, Self-like parts. Caring parts usually align with the child and polarize with the parents, which means they contribute to more polarization between the child and the parents.

The therapist can form a relationship with their caring part by noticing it, noticing how they feel toward it, befriending it, and inquiring about its fears, as we do in IFS therapy. This therapist learned that their concerned part was worried about Philip feeling alone and being labeled a troublemaker by the adults around him. It enjoyed Philip and couldn't understand why no one else saw his strengths. It thought Philip deserved to be loved and appreciated, not blamed. The part wanted to help both Philip and his mother understand him.

"Ask your caring part what it's afraid would happen if it couldn't help Philip see how much he has to offer other people?"

"It doesn't even want to begin thinking about that! Its job is to help kids. If I can't do that … What an awful feeling."

"Is it okay to check in to that awful feeling?" I asked.

"What would I be? I'd have no value. I'd be worthless."

With this statement, the therapist realized that the caring part was protecting them from feeling worthless by trying to protect Philip. That is, by listening to its motives, the therapist was acknowledging their caring part and its motives. This relational act facilitates unblending. If you see someone for who they are, they're clearly not you. The more the therapist's parts unblend, the more Self-energy the therapist has. After the therapist recognized and understood the protective part and got a glimpse of the exile who was being protected, they had some options. They could choose to explore the exile, check around for other parts, consider how their exile and its protectors might impact Philip and/or his mother, or they could shift to a more theoretical discussion about how to proceed with Philip and his mother. This therapist felt sufficiently unblended to be curious about how their caring protector was impacting Philip's mother.

"Sometimes it's easiest to start by letting the part blend a little. Think about Philip's mom, let this part blend, and see what you notice."

"Yikes, it's pretty intense! The 'caring' (using air quotes) part is angry at her. It's all geared up for a fight with Mom."

"Is it okay to stick with this and see what comes next?"

"Yep. The part has lots of ideas about how she could help Philip, but feels rejected by Mom, who always says either that my suggestions won't work or she'll try it, but she never does."

As the therapist talked, I scanned for reactions from my parts and used them as a template to guess how the mother's parts might react to the therapist's angry energy. "Anything else?" I asked.

"No, that's it."

"As I was listening to you, I pretended I was Philip's mother. Are you okay hearing how my parts reacted?"

"Sure."

"Right off I knew you cared about Philip. That felt good to some of my parts. But others felt scared and jealous. Like, what if Philip ends up liking you more than me? Then I started to imagine what you think about me. At first, I imagined positive things and felt a little hopeful. But then I felt afraid that I wouldn't be able to do what you want me to do. That made me feel like I can't do anything right. But it was too embarrassing to say any of that to you, so I decided to just say yes and avoid you … How are you doing? Was that hard to hear?"

"It was in a way, but I also got clear that I don't intend her to feel that way at all!"

"I know! That's the thing about caring parts. They have so much love and they're trying to help, but they end up landing on people in unintended ways. Can we shift back inside and notice the caring part?" I asked.

The therapist nodded.

"Okay. Ask it to unblend and be with you. Appreciate what it's been trying to do. Listen to its ideas, it probably has some really good ones. And see if it's open to letting you speak for it with Philip's mother."

Speaking *for* rather than *from* parts is a crucial concept in IFS. Parts are attached to their agendas, and when they blend (when we are speaking *from* the part) we can affect others in unintended ways, as Philip's mother's protector affected the therapist's caring part in an unintended way. However, when parts unblend (when we are able to speak *for* the part) and the Self is in the lead, we can share thoughts, concerns, ideas, and so on without being attached to a particular outcome. This approach invites parts rather than trying to control them. While my parts' reactions were not identical to the mother's, noticing and reviewing them helped the therapist's caring part unblend so the therapist could see what the part intended to accomplish. If the therapist was able to be more Self-led and less polarized with Philip's mother, their conversation would go more smoothly.

After this consultation, the therapist was able to make a small repair with the mother, which she described in the next consultation session.

"I was able to talk with Philip's mother and I think the conversation went as well as possible. I told her that I care about Philip and I am aware of a big desire to help him. I wondered how my intensity felt to her, and I invited her feedback. To my surprise, she said she was intimidated by me and that she just couldn't do the things I suggested. We had a good talk about that. Then I explained IFS to her in a different way, which she seemed to take in and she thanked me. However, her parts who were eager for Philip to change quickly had already decided to take Philip to a different therapist. I feel okay about that because we ended on a good note. I said come back if the new therapist doesn't work out."

This outcome illustrates a common complication for child therapy and child therapy consultation. Children tend to be referred by parents or teachers who want to change something about the child. In Philip's case, his mother, teachers, and after school providers all had parts who urgently wanted to stop Philip from feeling anxious and being aggressive. Their managers wanted his exiles to stop feeling their feelings and his firefighters to stop doing their jobs. This was the need and agenda of their managers. Since firefighters don't quit until exiles are unburdened, they were bound to be disappointed. Philip's need, in contrast, was to form a relationship with a Self-led therapist in which his parts felt welcomed, especially his aggressive firefighter part. If that part felt safe enough, the therapist would be able to help Philip unburden the exiles who fueled the firefighter's aggression, and everyone would be able to relax.

Polarizations and Alignments In and Between Systems

As well as knowing our own parts and how they are likely to show up in consultation, we also need to expect that polarizations and alignments will develop within and across systems and know how to help. Parts have an intricate social web in which some get into conflict and others join forces. This creates a tentative balance but does not achieve harmony for the system. As a result, polarizations and alignments are critical aspects of human relationships and a foundational concept in the IFS therapy.

In the first edition of *Internal Family Systems Therapy*, Schwartz borrows the metaphor from Paul Watzlawick and his colleagues to explain this concept. Imagine

> two sailors hanging out of either side of a sailboat in order to steady it: the more the one leans overboard, the more the other has to compensate for the instability created by the other's attempts at stabilizing the boat.
>
> (Watzlawick, Weakland, & Fisch, 1974, p. 36, as cited in Schwartz, 1995, p. 42)

While polarizations and alliances achieve their own kind of balance, when vulnerable parts have been exiled, they work in opposition to each other continually, forestalling the client from accessing any sense of ease or harmony. For example, let's say the child has inner polarizations in which protectors behave in opposite ways. One uses anger to protect a wounded exile, while the other uses compliance. These parts impact people around the child (parents, therapist, and even consultant) by eliciting parts in these other systems who either polarize or align. One or both parents may have parts who dislike the child's angry protector and polarize with it, or who favor the compliant protector and align with it. The inner system of the child also impacts the consultant and the therapist, as do the polarizations and alignments between the parents and the child.

Consultation is effective when the consultant is able to help the therapist unblend from their parts. To do that, the consultant starts by tuning in and unblending from any of their own parts who have mobilized in response to the child's protectors, the parents' reactivity, or the therapist's parts. As always in IFS, consultation involves nesting systems and parallel processing. If you cleave to the goal of Self-leadership by helping your parts unblend and healing your own exiles, you'll find you can navigate with more clarity than you might expect given the potential complexities of consulting to multiple embedded systems.

Lily

Lily was a 16-year-old girl who binged and purged about three or four times a week. She was referred to the therapist after an inpatient hospitalization, which had been requested by her parents. Lily was very bright and an excellent student. She appeared to be easy going, kind, and gentle. Lily had been seeing the therapist for nine months and was able to communicate with her own parts. That therapy had begun to develop relationships with some of her protectors, but the bingeing and purging still happened three or four times a week.

"Which parts has Lily connected with?" I asked.

"She's met an easy-going part that's around a lot. We've also touched base with an anxious one, and we're starting to get to know one that's pretty angry. We haven't gotten to the one that binges or purges though, which worries me a little," the therapist replied.

Since I took this last statement to be the concern of a part, I asked it directly, without stopping to clarify whether it was a part and, if it was, without helping the part to unblend, "What worries you about that?"

"I think we're doing good work, but it's going a lot slower than I want. She won't go inside every time, maybe just once out of every three or four sessions. Otherwise, she talks about feeling judged or watched by her parents and then wanting to binge more."

As the therapist talked, I noticed a part who felt urgent about helping Lily and also a part who felt helpless and trapped when the therapist described the parents watching Lily. I wondered if Lily felt this and asked the therapist, "Did she say how it feels when she's watched?"

"She said she feels boxed in and hates it."

"When she feels boxed in, how does she react to her parents?"

"Sometimes she gets mad but doesn't tell them why. Sometimes she leaves the house. And sometimes she binges."

"Okay. What else do you need me to know? And, if you want, let's talk about your parts, too."

"My parts are polarized! Sometimes I think we're doing great work and things are starting to change for Lily. Then, when I hear about the bingeing, I think I'm not doing enough to push her. Before I meet with Lily's parents, I bounce back and forth between those two feelings. When I meet with them, I get stuck thinking I should do more, so she'll stop bingeing."

"Tell me about that."

"Her parents love her and want to help. They're smart and analytical and can't understand why Lily won't just stop bingeing and purging. They're so anxious they keep asking me when she will stop. I've explained about protectors and exiles, and they're trying hard to accept my assurances that it will stop eventually. But they watch Lily like a couple of hawks."

As I listened, I felt compassion for the parents and their daughter. I also felt a desire to fix this situation and give them what they longed for.

"How does that affect you?" I asked.

"I want to help them, but I feel stuck in the middle. It seems the only way I can help the parents is to stop Lily from bingeing and purging. But when that part of me takes over, I push Lily and she shuts down. Then I think Lily could do this if she weren't feeling watched and judged, but I can't get the parents to stop. Help!"

"How would you like to approach this? We can start with your parts or anything else that feels helpful."

"I need to get clear about what's going on between me, Lily, and her parents."

"It might help, then, to think about this in terms of polarizations and alignments. Some of your parts are likely either polarized or aligned with Lily and/or her parents, and the same is true of their parts. Let's start with Lily. Which of her parts do you notice?"

"So, there are the bingeing and purging parts we haven't met. Then there's the easy-going one, the anger, and the anxiety. I'm not sure about exiles … Well, Lily describes feeling trapped when she's watched and judged. That's probably an exile."

"Let's track what happens between Lily and her parents after Lily binges and purges. What happens after the parents discover Lily has binged and purged?"

"Neither of them actually says anything about it. The mom reports getting very anxious and trying to hide it by being 'manically supportive,' as Lily calls it, and pretending nothing has happened. This doesn't feel like support to Lily. She senses her mother's intense anxiety. Meanwhile, Dad disappears into his study and doesn't engage with either of them."

"Let's start with Lily's reaction to her mother. Has she said anything about that?"

"It's sad, really. Lily's gut reaction is to try and take care of her mother. She can't bear her anxiety."

"What else?"

"This is where that angry part shows up, although she never expresses the anger directly. This part thinks stuff like, 'Aren't you supposed to take care of me? Why do I always have to take care of you?'"

"Who is the angry part polarized with?"

"Well, Lily's critic, I guess. It tells her, 'This is your fault, Lily. If you weren't so awful, your mother wouldn't feel this way.' This critic makes her feel hollow in the stomach."

"And how does Lily react to her dad withdrawing?"

"Again, it's sad. When Dad withdraws, Lily's critic immediately activates and lists everything wrong with her. If she just weren't so − fill in the blank − her dad wouldn't need to get away from her. So, she ends up feeling judged by her own critic as well as by her dad."

"I'm guessing that activates the hollow feeling in her stomach, too."

"Yes."

"Now let's switch to you. Is that okay? What comes up in you around these interactions between Lily and her parents? Start wherever feels right."

"I'll start with Lily. First, I always notice a protector that loves Lily and wants to help her. It feels connected to her and doesn't want to fail her."

"Does this part push you to move faster with Lily?"

"Absolutely! And there's another part that pushes even harder because it's anxious about the long-term physical effects of bingeing and purging. When it takes over, I'm afraid she'll die. That part wants her to stop the eating disorder right now."

"That makes sense."

"Then the part that wants to explain everything to Lily is always around. Her parents have the same belief that understanding will stop her from bingeing and purging. When Lily won't talk parts, I get into explaining."

"What is your explaining part trying to protect in you?"

"Earlier, when I mentioned Lily's hollow feeling, I noticed a twinge of the same in me."

"Good observing. Are you open to focusing on the parts of you who activate with the parents?"

"Sure. I never saw this before, but I think my parts might be very similar to theirs. I notice a part that really likes the parents and doesn't want to let them down. It wants to spare them the pain of watching Lily endangering herself this way, and it wants to help Lily stop bingeing and purging sooner rather than later. Another one shares their anxiety about Lily and gets amped up when I feel the anxiety of either Mom or Dad."

"That all makes sense. Anything else?"

"I also have an intellectual part that tries to educate Lily and spends a lot of time talking with the parents. And, when I feel like I'm not doing enough, I start to notice that hollow feeling in my stomach again."

"Do you want to spend time with any of those parts here?"

"No, I can do that in my therapy. Let's make a plan for my work with Lily."

"Of course. First, being aware of your parts will help you to help them unblend before and during sessions, especially the ones who think it would be helpful for Lily to stop bingeing and purging immediately. While the pushing parts are trying to help you, the ones in Lily who binge and purge will just believe you want to get rid of them. If they don't feel welcome, you and Lily won't get any traction with them."

"I understand."

"Our protectors create unintended consequences. As the polarization between your parts and Lily's parts relaxes, I'm confident she'll be more willing to go deeper in sessions. The same is true with her parents. As you have more Self-energy, you'll be curious towards them rather than wanting to rescue them, which will help them get curious about their own protectors and their impact on their daughter."

Once the therapist was more Self-led, the therapy experience changed for both Lily and her parents. Over the next several months, Lily found and healed the part who felt hollow, and the bingeing and purging parts calmed down and eventually stopped. Meanwhile, the therapist helped Lily's parents notice and unblend their anxious parts, which decreased their anxiety at home with Lily and increased their curiosity about their relationships with her. In response, Lily's protectors settled down, and she became more curious about her inner life.

Lily's case highlights the challenge for IFS therapists and consultants, especially those who work with children, of distinguishing between caring, helping parts in the therapist and the therapist's Self. The energy of caring parts can feel like Self-energy, but it has a very different impact, as Lily's case illustrates. If you wonder whether a consultee (therapist) is leading from Self-energy, notice how their client's parts respond to the caring interaction. Lily's protective system was "allergic to" the caring parts of her therapist. A negative response like this tells you quickly and definitively that a caring part is in the driver's seat rather than the therapist's Self. In fact, Lily's system had the same reaction to any caring parts, whether those of the therapist or her parents. Parents care, family physicians care, educators care, therapists care, and so on. We have therapist parts who are specifically trained in various ways of caring. A significant part of my 20 plus years practicing IFS has been devoted to discovering and distinguishing between my caring parts and my Self. I recommend the same investigation to all IFS therapists.

Conclusion

This chapter illustrates how child therapy consultants can help therapists apply the principles of IFS across multiple systems. First and foremost, the consultant notices how their parts react to the therapist's story and offers this information to the therapist as a clue to the motives and feelings of others in the therapeutic system, which consists of parents, child, and therapist. Throughout consultation, the therapist is in charge of what to focus on. They may choose to delve into the reactions of their parts, which will usually include polarizations and alignments. In order to look at polarizations and alignments within and between any or all of the systems involved, both the therapist and the consultant will need to help their parts unblend. Finally, the therapist may choose to ask technical questions and discuss theory.

IFS child therapy consultation is multi-layered and, for me, immensely rewarding. It gives me the opportunity to help therapists transform the lives of children and their caretakers. At the same time, I benefit personally because every consultation session gives me a bird's-eye view of my internal system as it interacts with other systems. From the perspective of the Self, I always make new internal discoveries and become a better therapist and, I believe, a better person. Just as time and practice are essential for improving in the role of therapist, time and practice are essential for growing and improving in the role of IFS consultant. I'm much better at consulting now than I was when I started. My parts trust me, unblend willingly, and let me lead. I encourage you to jump in, practice, and experience the same rewards.

Note

1 I thank Martha Sweezy for her editorial help.

References

Gomez, A. M., & Krause, P. K. (2013). EMDR therapy and the use of Internal Family Systems strategies with children. In A. M. Gomez (Ed.), *EMDR therapy and adjunct approaches with children: Complex trauma, attachment, and dissociation.* (pp. 299–319). Springer Press.

Krause, P. K. (2013). IFS with children and adolescents. In M. Sweezy & E. L. Ziskind (Eds.), *Internal Family Systems therapy: New dimensions* (pp. 35–54). Routledge.

Schwartz, R. C. (1995). *Internal Family Systems therapy.* The Guilford Press.

5 Consultation for the IFIO Therapist

Ann E. Drouilhet

I am being observed, and it is uncomfortable. Together on Zoom, the IFIO training staff is practicing the skill of providing a demonstration to training participants, of one of the basic protocols offered by IFIO. I love and trust my colleagues, and parts of me even welcome their feedback. And yet my heart rate is elevated, and I can feel protector parts start to activate as they consider fight, flight, or freeze. And of course, as is always the case, I now have less access to Self-energy, especially curiosity and creativity. Just like what happens to the therapists for whom I provide IFIO consultation. A good reminder to keep me humble and compassionate.

Introduction

This chapter offers descriptions of common issues and dilemmas in providing consultation for clinicians who are using Intimacy From the Inside Out (IFIO), which is the application of IFS to couple therapy. I provide a brief overview of the theory and practice of IFIO, and I discuss the role of the consultant in teaching methodology and in helping clinicians track their own parts. Anonymized case examples of clinicians triggered in working with couples and of how consultants might get triggered in the work are included, together with suggestions for returning to Self-leadership. Note that I am a White, middle-aged, heterosexual, cisgender woman, keenly aware of the privilege of being middle class and the advantages that my race, education, and financial security have afforded me. The clinicians who seek me out for consultation have similar demographics and primarily work with White clients, some with gender and sexual diversity. In my own clinical practice and consultation, I regularly reflect on my biases – implicit and explicit – and their impact on my formulations and interventions. In every conversation we have, I encourage consultees to do the same. This does not detract from the applicability of IFIO to working with couples in circumstances different to my own and who identify very differently.

DOI: 10.4324/9781003044864-5

Intimacy From the Inside Out

The application of IFS to working with couples has been articulated by Toni Herbine-Blank on her website (toniherbineblank.com) and YouTube channel as well as in two books: *Intimacy from the Inside Out: Courage and Compassion in Couple Therapy* (Herbine-Blank et al., 2016) and *Internal Family Systems Couple Therapy Skills Manual* (Herbine-Blank & Sweezy, 2021). This chapter highlights the unique qualities of this model of couple therapy.

Therapists interested in the study and practice of IFIO will be well served to have first completed at least the Level 1 IFS training, which is offered worldwide and taught by IFS Institute trainers. That training explicitly teaches the theory and method for working with individual clients using the IFS model. Concepts from the IFS model that are especially relevant to practicing IFIO include:

- Non-pathological multiplicity of mind (parts);
- Self (inner wisdom);
- Appreciating the positive intention of all protector parts;
- A paradigm of healing between Self and parts;
- Making a U-turn (first being curious about one's own reactivity before focusing on the behavior and motivations of the other);
- Unblending (inner differentiation of Self from parts and parts from parts, which is essential for self-regulation);
- Attuning to sensations in the body (the body is a resource for tracking one's emotional system);
- The understanding that "we are them" (the idea that therapists experience and struggle with the same dilemmas as their clients);
- Recognizing the close pairing between protectors and the parts being protected (understanding that the extremity of protectors is driven by exile vulnerability); and
- People live in polarizations inside and out, and a partner may project the qualities of a disavowed part of their own internal polarization onto their partner. The partner, due to their own internal polarization, usually unconsciously, "accepts" and enacts the projected qualities of the partner's part.

The assumptions of IFIO include:

- What is possible in the work with an individual is possible with a couple, such as deep healing inside and out;
- Inner security of the individual supports relational bonding;
- The more partners are differentiated internally and interpersonally, the healthier their attachment;
- Affect regulation (unblending) is key to the effective negotiation of needs;

- The model is experiential and process oriented; and
- Self-regulation and co-regulation support each other and affect neurobiology (Cozolino, 2006; Ecker et al., 2012; Seigel, 2007).

The goals of IFIO include:

- To shift attention away from one's partner to one's inner feelings, impulses, and patterns of responding;
- To decrease reactivity and to increase self-empowerment, which leads to more choices of how to speak and listen;
- To increase Self-leadership;
- To change the conversation;
- To skillfully repair a rupture, both minor and major; and
- To jointly envision a new way of relating.

The IFIO Roadmap

The protocols taught in the Basic IFIO training (see Figure 5.1), include first building a therapeutic alliance by developing safety and trust between the couple and the therapist, then identifying the repeated patterns of their conflict (tracking sequences), teaching and supporting each member of the couple to recognize and unblend from their protector parts (differentiating), doing intrapsychic or individual work in the presence of the other as appropriate, facilitating the skill of speaking on behalf of parts and listening from Self (courageous communication), making a meaningful repair, and envisioning a different future. Although these protocols are taught in a linear fashion, we remind trainees that these are non-linear protocols, and the IFIO therapist may return repeatedly to protocols they were using earlier in therapy (for example, returning to tracking a sequence between the couple if reactivity re-emerges when starting to set up courageous communication). The gift of these protocols is that they provide a "roadmap" for IFIO therapists, allowing them to know at any moment in the therapy what they are doing and why – even if it doesn't seem to be going well in the moment. This supports the therapist's experience of "holding their seat," even with highly reactive couples where one or both partners are hyperaroused or hypoaroused.

The Role of the IFIO Consultant

Herbine-Blank et al. (2016, p. 85) remind us that, "Couple therapists must navigate some extremely complex situations. To do so effectively, we look inward first, developing and maintaining solid internal connections and discovering what's happening with our parts when we feel stuck." The IFIO consultant contracts with the consulting therapist for a regular inquiry into what they are noticing in their heart, mind, and body as a therapy with

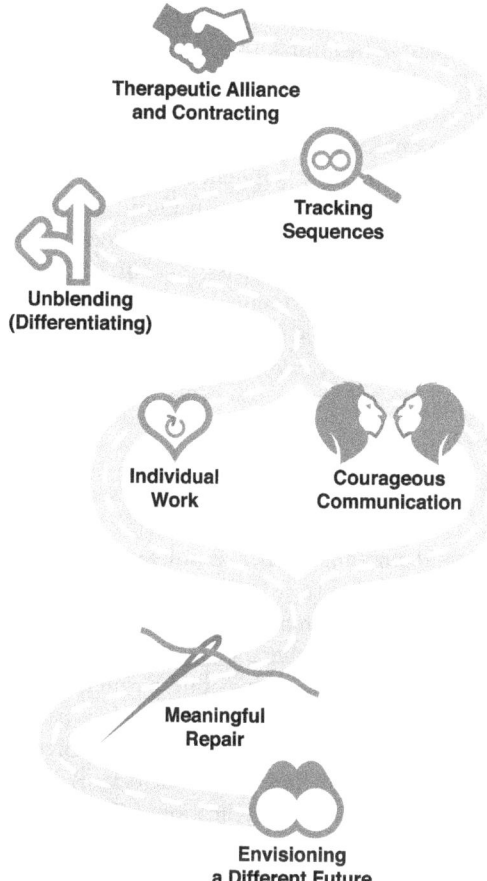

Figure 5.1 An IFIO Roadmap
Source: Adapted and used by permission of Toni Herbine-Blank

a couple evolves. The consultation contract also includes direction and input from the consultant regarding the consultee's skills and use of the tools taught in IFIO, which can be thought of as "therapist parts."

Contracting

As in any good therapy in which the therapist initiates an agreement or contract for the goals of the work and regularly revisits the goals and agreement, the IFIO consultant has a similar role with the consultee. It can be tempting for the seasoned consultant and consultee to forgo this part of the conversation – the negotiating of a consultation contract – as if the fact of their long experience allows both to assume that there is a mutual understanding of the nature of *this* relationship that doesn't really need to be articulated. I have parts that regretfully, in retrospect, have allowed such assumptions to dominate. This mistake becomes painfully obvious when the consultee gets triggered, especially in response to feedback from the consultant, and has the experience of vulnerability (which often is accompanied by shame). An agreement/contract provides a plan to help guide how the pair will talk together about what happened between them and how both will make a U-turn to make room for curiosity about and toward their reactions. In addition to clarifying how often to meet and for how long as well as payment and cancellation policies, a contract/agreement for consultation includes a record of the trainee's goals, growing edges, and parts that get triggered. It also includes a commitment to regularly evaluate the consultation relationship: what is working and what needs to be modified.

Expectations and Offerings

As a consultant, I provide guidance on how to present a case and formulate clinical questions; I teach through demonstrations, role-play, visualization, and video recording; I encourage the consultee to speak about their formulations and ideas for interventions; and I welcome the many polarizations that regularly show up in the therapist while making clinical decisions. I explain that it is common for a therapist is get triangulated with a couple (Bowen, 1978; Minuchin, 1974), such as one partner wanting the therapist to side with them in a judgment against the other partner. I invite the consultee to be curious about their formative experiences in earlier triangular relationships (especially in their family of origin) and their protective parts that originated from these complications. For example, a therapist, who as a child took on the responsibility of keeping their parents together, might find themself trying to convince one or both members of the couple of the merits of their partner. The sense of urgency in this convincing behavior may be fueled by the fear of the therapist's exile that if the couple breaks up, it is the therapist's fault and evidence of not being good enough.

I also allow regular time for the consultee to develop their skill at tracking their own protectors and exiles throughout the work with the couple. I remind the consultee that, as consultant, I also am tracking my emotional system as I engage in the complex process of offering consultation to them. I do this with the hope that sharing my experience reduces any unhelpful sense of hierarchy and supports a spirit of collaboration.

I make a strong pitch to every consultee to video their sessions and present them for consultation. Watching a session together allows for a more accurate understanding of what is happening in the session and for feedback to be more relevant for both technical recommendations and tracking the parts of the therapist. Self-report is limited and constrained by protector parts who, mostly unconsciously, are unable to re-present what happens in a session in a meaningful way. This recommendation is often met with parts that agree in theory but are polarized with parts fearing exposure and possible shame, holding concerns about clients' reactions to being recorded, and worrying about managing the technology involved in making a recording. Hearing and validating these protectors may help them trust our process and be willing to record sessions even if some discomfort persists.

Without the advantage of our watching the consultee's videos together, I have a part who worries that my feedback is not accurate or useful. This worried part distracts me from careful listening and can trigger an impatient part who puts me at risk of compromising my attunement to the consultee's dilemma. When I notice these protectors and appreciate their intention to help me be responsive to the needs of the consultee, they relax and allow me to stay open and curious even when the consultee provides only a verbal description of the treatment.

Offering the consultee a recording of the consultation session is valuable for teaching and learning. Video recording role-play allows both of us to examine the pros and cons of different interventions at a choice-point in a session. The opportunity for the consultee to observe the consultants' relative comfort with being videotaped can strengthen their trust and safety in the consultation relationship. Working with the trailheads revealed by parts who get triggered by watching themselves on video deepens the confidence, courage, and skill development of both consultee and consultant.

Common Challenges for Less Experienced IFIO Therapists

Several common and predictable challenges emerge when the consultee is learning to apply the theory and method of IFIO couple therapy. Some consultees find that working with (unblending from) their uncertain or reactive parts once or twice is sufficient to continue from Self. Others who continue to get stuck can benefit from a deeper dive into their system (see Chapter 6, Herbine-Blank et al., 2016) to understand and heal the protector parts and their corresponding exiles, which frees them up to apply their IFIO skills in clearer and newer ways. The consultant and consultee should discuss how much exploration is appropriate for the consultation relationship and which trailheads could be addressed in the consultee's personal therapy. This negotiation will be different with each consultee. Most important is for the consultant to be mindful of such tender territory and not launch into an inner exploration without explicit agreement with the consultee and their parts. A current consultee offered the following feedback: "You are extremely compassionate but purposeful in helping me to notice when I'm leading from a part rather than from my Self. Without your courage to address that, my parts would keep on keeping on in those same ways."

Straying from the IFIO Roadmap

A poignant example of the common challenge of staying on the IFIO roadmap is demonstrated in the work of a consultee, Robert. Robert is a middle-aged, White, cisgender male who made a career change from computer programming after the loss of a child to cancer. Although new to psychotherapy, he was very influenced and inspired by the couple therapy that he and his wife received during his child's illness and death. As consultant, I notice that Robert seems to be abandoning the IFIO protocols in favor of more directive and advice-giving interventions. My first intervention is to negotiate with Robert about his availability to notice when he is no longer using the IFIO methodology. My observation that he has "gone off-piste" comes as a bit of a shock for Robert and evokes parts ashamed of not using the model correctly and anxious that he will never be an effective IFIO therapist. I respond by validating the concerns of those parts and by inviting Robert to be curious with me about which parts choose to give advice instead of staying with the IFIO method. Robert discovers a protector who feels impatient with the couple's progress and worried that *any* conflict between the partners is proof that they are still suffering. This part cannot tolerate the possibility that the couple is in pain and feels desperately responsible for alleviating their suffering quickly, especially since the couple is paying him "out of pocket." The part believes that Robert doesn't deserve to be paid if the couple is still struggling. This part stays blended with Robert despite the couple regularly telling him how much improvement they are experiencing and how grateful they are for his work with them. With additional inquiry, this protector shows Robert the more vulnerable part of him whom it believes it is protecting. With the blessing of the protector, Robert connects with a young exile burdened with the belief that if Robert is not "helping," then he, the exile, is not good enough and not worthy of love. When Robert makes an intention to work with this young part in his individual therapy, the protector is reassured enough to trust Robert to come back to the principles and methodology of IFIO. While this protector had been scrambling to find any intervention that might work with the couple, it now gives space for Robert to be curious with them about their remaining cycles of conflict that catch them only occasionally.

Becoming Triggered by Clients' Reactions

Parts of the IFIO therapist who are afraid of certain clients and couples get triggered by clients' protectors, who express, among other things, disappointment in the therapy ("We aren't making progress"); disagreement with something the therapist said ("That's not right"), accusations ("You seem to be taking her side and see me as the problem"), hostility and discouragement ("What's the point?"), or anger (expressed indirectly with sighs and eye rolls).

Kay, a consultee in her 40s and a seasoned couple therapist new to IFIO, is repeatedly concerned about a client's reaction to her being several minutes late to the session. She agrees with the client that she should be on time and accepts that her lateness feels like disrespect to the client. And she is aware of an exile in her system who believes that the client's anger is further proof of how bad she is. Her guilt and shame contribute to a sense of dread in anticipation of the next session. She notices a protector who both holds her back from inviting the client to tell her more about her reaction to Kay's lateness and tries to steel Kay for an anticipated next attack. As a result, Kay leads with an overly solicitous and complimentary part who constrains her from getting curious about the burdens carried by the client's protector (*I can't tolerate disrespect*) and exile (*I don't matter*). Kay's protectors also restrain her from checking with the other member of the couple about their experience and the impact of Kay's lateness on them – as though parts of Kay assume that both members of the couple feel the same way. With deeper exploration, Kay becomes aware of a part of her that also feels undervalued and even taken advantage of by the couple. This part tells her: *Yeah, but what about the fact that I frequently extend the session (especially when they are in the middle of a difficult conversation) by 20 minutes at no extra cost when I don't have an appointment following theirs?* And: *What about how I find additional time in my overly booked schedule when they are in a "crisis"?* And: *What about when I return their phone calls and emails within hours of hearing from them?* In summary, if *any* client is triggered by something Kay does, an exile believes it is her fault, knows she is bad, and should be ashamed. The dominant protector that keeps Kay feeling and acting small, questioning her competence as a therapist, and preparing (and sometimes wishing) for the clients to terminate the therapy is polarized with a part that feels judgment and disdain in response to the client's complaints. The guilt that Kay feels in response to these thoughts is assuaged by her manager going "the extra mile" with the hope that this will prevent the clients from reacting negatively to her tardiness.

As safety and trust have evolved in the consultation relationship, Kay has increasingly been able to disclose how frequently parts get scared of certain clients. This has allowed for an exploration of polarized protectors – one who feels responsible for a client's negative feelings in contrast to a part who believes it is an injustice to her hard work if a client complains. Kay has a renewed interest in helping the exile (a trailhead for individual therapy) to receive the attention it needs in order to feel safe with Kay, even when a client's reactive parts "attack" her. As her protectors witness the relationship Kay is building with the exile, they are beginning to trust Self and make room for Kay to move toward the client's angry firefighters without Kay blaming herself for being late or for making any other "mistake" that triggers a member of the couple into directing "an attack" at Kay or at their partner.

Creating the Couple Therapy Contract

Clarifying the goals of therapy with a couple is frequently missed by both newer and more seasoned clinicians. Complaints and criticisms by each partner toward the other can confuse the goals and purpose of the therapy, especially when the therapist does not explicitly ask, "Is this what you want to work on in your therapy with me?" Asking this question (or a variation on it) in the first sessions and regularly throughout the therapy helps the therapist decide what interventions to use at particular moments and helps the therapist keep an eye on any agenda their own parts might have for the couple. I have been intrigued (and dismayed) at how frequently consultees struggle with asking the question of a couple: "What do you want from the therapy?" This seems especially true the more complicated the case and the more fierce the protectors – all the more reason to be reviewing with the couple every session their goals for the therapy and for the current session in service of their larger goals.

For example, it is important to make an explicit connection for the couple between engaging in a U-turn and each partner's deep yearning to be heard and understood by their partner. The couple's fierce protectors may then be willing to reveal the burdens that hold them back from allowing the therapist to support accessing curiosity about what is triggering in their system, which requires the rescue of the protective system. Gently and firmly, IFIO therapists remind protectors that they can help by trusting the Self of the client. That way, the partners can receive what they most want, which usually is acceptance, safety, and love, both internally and externally.

It can be difficult for some IFIO consultees to explore on a regular basis a couple's goals for therapy. It can be equally difficult to be asked about this in consultation and not have an answer. For consultee Joanne, my asking the questions "What does the couple say they want from therapy?" and "What did the couple want to work on during that particular session?" evokes strong feelings. Joanne hears from parts of her who say, *I should know this* (shame) and *What does it mean about me that I keep forgetting to ask?* (fear). In our exploration, Joanne considers that not asking is the strategy of her part who believes she should know without having to explicitly ask. This protector part is working very hard to convince the couple of Joanne's competence and pushes Joanne to quickly move on to protocols, such as tracking sequences or courageous communication, before clarifying and confirming the couple's goals for the therapy or the session. Joanne hears from this protector that it believes that the couple will not have confidence in her ability to help them if she asks them for clarification, and she will expose that she doesn't know something that this part believes she should know. This part anticipates the couple will be annoyed and impatient with her, which will be wounding to a young, vulnerable part who, like Kay's part, is burdened with beliefs about not being good enough and that it won't be valued. Joanne tracks her early experiences with caregivers who would chastise her for not anticipating their needs and validates how and when a young part (an exile) became burdened with fears of not being good enough and anticipating rejection. She then understands how a protector part got its job of quickly moving into "helping" the couple before

Joanne has all of the information she needs to make an informed decision about what next to offer the couple in service of their goals for the therapy.

IFIO Emphasizes Process Over Content: Protectors Shield Exiles

IFIO is a model of couple therapy that emphasizes process over content. Of course the therapist has to initially hear the story, including the history of grievances. Like in IFS therapy, storytelling parts are asked to soften back in order to explore parts who repeat unsuccessful strategies to try to satisfy vulnerable longings. As the hopes and fears of each partner are understood and validated, the IFIO therapist offers the couple an invitation to learn the skills of speaking on behalf of their parts and listening from Self. In this way each of them can effectively negotiate their needs with less reactive frustration inside themselves and from the other, leading them to discover the possibility of deeper intimacy. Especially for therapists trained in other models of couple therapy, emphasizing process over content is a paradigm shift that is very appealing and often challenging to stick with. After the initial phase of politeness between couple and therapist, the couple lays bare the true nature of their conflict as their protectors fight and parry in their attempts to protect vulnerable exiles and get their needs met. When this escalation starts to alarm the exiles of the therapist, getting triangulated into the couple's relationship is a common result. Some therapist's protectors will often try to shield the therapist's vulnerable exiles by getting engaged in the content of the conflict. Other therapist protector behaviors include feeling an urgency (often not conscious) to "fix" the couple, which often means trying to keep them together; dropping curiosity in favor of solutions (e.g., teaching communication skills); and resorting to interventions promoted by other models of couple therapy (e.g., negotiating behavioral contracts). The effective application of the IFIO protocols helps the therapist to keep the issues *between* the couple, inviting them to become increasingly aware of their patterns of interaction and the internal processes that contribute to their maintenance. But becoming proficient at employing IFIO protocols requires patience and perseverance and an understanding of and belief in what they offer the couple (and therapist) – all of which comes with practice and consultation.

When sticking with a protocol is challenging, I first confirm the level of understanding of the goals of the protocol and then assess the consultees' skill of application. Watching a video of a therapy session or role-playing aspects of the session will clarify misunderstandings and gaps in effective use of the method. Then I invite the therapist to extend curiosity to parts that may hold them back from using the protocols as designed; my intention is to make it safe for parts who are not fully on board with using the protocols to reveal themselves. A consultee, Raymond, has recently discovered an exile who is burdened with fear of being seen as incompetent by the couple when they complain that they are not making progress. He makes the connection between the exile, vigilant for any sign that the couple is mad at him, and the protectors steering him away from using the protocols (U-turn, unblending, speaking on behalf of parts), believing they will trigger more reactivity in the couple, thus putting his exile at risk (*I'm unworthy*). In these moments of anxiety, Raymond's protectors believe they are responsible for the couple changing, for preventing conflict, and for explaining the clients to themselves and each other. These are common strategies of well-meaning protectors who are dedicated to burdened exiles, believe this is an emergency, and can't tolerate the risk associated with sticking with the protocol. These protectors hold Raymond back from effectively applying the IFIO methods even though other parts are committed to doing so. Exploration of this polarity and a commitment to building a Self-to-part relationship with his exile have increased Raymond's confidence. He has a sense now of his ability to "hold his seat" even when a couple is directing their distress about therapy not helping, or not helping fast enough, toward him.

The Importance of Not Relying Solely on Therapist Self-Report

As previously recommended, watching videos of the consultee's work with couples allows for seeing strategies of therapist protector parts that the therapist is usually unable to self-report. These behaviors include: talking too much or too little, a reluctance to interrupt, not tolerating silence, and not recognizing when they are triggered and are intervening from a part. Concerns about the judgment of the consultant and worry that being triggered is evidence of not being a competent therapist often interfere with the consultee risking their work being directly observed. With recognition of the fear of these parts, the consultant's attunement to, compassion for, and courage to get to know these parts can make a difference and result in a consultee receiving direct feedback about their work, which has the potential to increase their skill and confidence in the long run.

The Consultant Gets Triggered

In addition to providing support and guidance to the consultee to track their own emotional system while working with any particular couple, as the IFIO consultant, I will be doing the same as the relationship evolves. As is true in any relationship, it is to be expected that the consultant will have reactions to the presentation of the consultee. These reactions, or protector parts, will call for care and attention from the consultant in service of remaining openhearted and Self-led while providing consultation.

Behaviors that might trigger me include when the consultee doesn't follow the guidelines agreed to for presenting a case and not having formulated specific questions to be addressed in the consultation. Understandably, sometimes a consultee is so overwhelmed by the complexity of a case that they may just need to talk for a while in service of gaining more clarity about both the couple and, perhaps even more important, the parts of them that are triggered and interfering with their ability to both present the case and formulate a question. Helping the consultee to recognize when this is happening and to welcome overwhelmed parts without shaming them is a skill of an effective consultant. Also triggering is when the consultee wants to talk at length about the couple's history, including lots of speculation about motivation and pathology, without pausing to consider where they are in the work and what protocols might be appropriate. This may alarm some parts of me as I am hoping to hear evidence of consistent adherence by the consultee to the basic premises of both IFS and IFIO. Recognizing one's own reactivity in the role of consultant and unblending from any alarmed or critical parts is essential for maintaining a consulting relationship that feels safe and helpful to the consultee. A Self-led consultant is able to help the consultee to bring curiosity to their part(s) who make assumptions and judgments about clients' intentions and motivations. Feedback from a different consultee speaks to this:

> You slow me down in a way that can frustrate me sometimes because my brain likes to go fast, but it's just as necessary for me to really slow down and think things through one part at a time as it is for the couples I work with. In doing that, I am able to get much clearer on whatever I'm talking about, and, maybe even more importantly, it gives me space to try to come to realizations myself. So, you're not spoon-feeding me answers, but you also don't leave me hanging if I'm stuck.

I can also get triggered when a consultee insists on filling the time with non-stop description of the case, barely pausing to let me even ask a question. The part triggered shows up in my body, creating a tension in my gut and jaw. It has a judgment about the consultee not showing enough deference to my expertise and wonders why she has even hired me if she isn't interested in what I have to say. I offer empathy and compassion to that part for its feelings of frustration. I ask what it might need to relax and let me find a way to bring curiosity, both in energy and word to the consultee, about what they might be noticing in the moment and any concerns they might be holding about the consultation. This part takes a deep breath, releases its grip on my body, and I can smile again.

Something similar happens for me when the consultee gives lip service to tracking her own emotional system. Having completed at least the basic IFIO training, the consultee is aware of the expectation that they will recognize and bring curiosity to their personal parts that are triggered. However, that doesn't guarantee that all parts are on board, and the consultee may need a firm but kind consultant to persist in asking the questions: "When you pause and go inside, what do you feel in your body?" "What are you hearing yourself say to yourself?" and "What is your first impulse?"

I can also get triggered and respond with confusion (that has an edge to it) when a consultee identifies a personal protector in one session, only to deny having done so in the next session. Using my breath, I ask my part to tell me about its reaction – "Tell me all about it." It is usually a part of mine that is trying so hard to get it right, wanting so earnestly to provide a good consultation, so that my younger, more vulnerable parts will feel reassured of their value. I let it know I understand and appreciate its dedication and its keen powers of observation. And I ask it to trust me to navigate a path with the consultee in which they get their needs met and the part and I feel satisfied with doing a good job. They then relax, which allows me to be curious (without the edge).

Recently, I found myself reacting to a consultee, Sivan, as she was describing a caretaking (my assessment) part that is insisting she meet with a client in her office, despite Sivan's concerns about COVID-19 and her own personal safety. I am immediately alarmed at this part's willingness to put Sivan in harm's way before exploring more thoroughly with the client his concerns about meeting online and the needs of his parts. As I notice a part of me reacting with protest and trying to convince her that she doesn't have to overextend herself to meet the client's demand, I become aware of my own caretaking part, the strategies it is using, and how it is creating a tension that feels like a power struggle between me and Sivan. I feel it in my chest and neck, and my energy is no longer collaborative but has taken on a hierarchical stance as part of me believes I need to tell her what to do. I can hear that this part of me feels justified in its approach given that it believes Sivan's caretaking part is going to put her at risk. As I lean into the sensations in my body and hear the concerns of this part, I am able to unblend and invite it to trust me to have a curious and compassionate conversation with Sivan about my concerns. Turning inward (a U-turn) allows me to return to Sivan with more openness and acceptance of the part insisting Sivan defer to the client's demand. As the tension between us dissipates and I am able to name and speak on behalf of my own caretaking part, Sivan becomes curious about her own caretaking part and aware that she has more choices than just giving into the client's "demand."

When It Goes Well

When it goes well, there is trust and safety for both the consultee and the consultant. The requirement in both the IFS and IFIO models that the therapists track their own emotional systems while tracking the clients' potentially renders therapists more vulnerable to feelings of inadequacy and shame when seeking out consultation. Not only is the therapist being asked to expose their professional work, but also to reveal their own thoughts and feelings (positive and negative) about their work and the possible origins of those reactions. All of which can leave the therapist feeling fraught with worry about the consultant's judgments and full of feelings of shame, although ultimately, if all goes well, such exposure and vulnerability results in the therapist becoming more effective. Similarly, this is an isomorphic process, and the consultant is also admonished to track her/his/their emotional system while interacting with the consultee.

To recap, when it goes well, there is a clarity in the consultation relationship around goals, which are revisited on a regular basis. The consultee is receptive to inquiries and willing to try something new, even if it is sticking more closely to the structure of a protocol that they thought they had already mastered. Also, there is a flow of feedback from the consultant, including support, encouragement, and recognition of how challenging couple therapy can be. Good IFIO consultation leads to the consultee having more choices of intervention and flexibility in how they use their own personhood together with a firmer sense of having found and held their seat, even in the face of couples whose suffering manifests as extreme reactivity.

References

Bowen, M. (1978). *Family therapy in clinical practice*. Jason Aronson.

Cozolino, L. (2006). *The neuroscience of human relationships: Attachment and the developing social brain*. Norton.

Ecker, B., Ticic, R., & Hulley, L. (2012). *Unlocking the emotional brain: Eliminating symptoms at their roots using memory reconsolidation*. Routledge.

Herbine-Blank, T., Kerpelman, D. M., & Sweezy, M., (2016). *Intimacy from the inside out: Courage and compassion in couple therapy*. Routledge.

Herbine-Blank, T. & Sweezy, M. (2021). *Internal Family Systems couple therapy skills manual: Healing relationships with Intimacy from the Inside Out*. PESI.

Minuchin, S. (1974). *Families and family therapy*. Harvard University Press.

Siegel, K. J. (2007). *The mindful brain: Reflection and attunement in the cultivation of well-being*. Norton.

6 Creating Access to IFS Training and Consultation for BIPOC Therapists

Black Therapists Rock Leads the Way

Tamala Floyd

This chapter details my experience as the Internal Family Systems (IFS) Consultant to Black Therapists Rock (BTR). As well as providing descriptions of the BTR organization and the role of the BTR-IFS Consultant, I discuss the relationship between BTR and the IFS Institute (IFS-I). Fictionalized case vignettes illuminate the work between consultant and consultee, and adaptations of the model to meet the needs of Black clients are presented.

Increasing Representation of Black Therapists in the IFS World

I am a licensed clinical social worker with over 25 years of clinical experience. I attended an IFS Level 1 training in January 2018. I was one of two Black people in attendance. Although a familiar occurrence for me, it is one I wish I didn't experience so frequently. The other Black woman was Deran Young, the founder and CEO of BTR. Deran and I did not know each other prior to this training. We happened to be assigned to the same reflection group (formerly called home group). This provided us the opportunity to get to know each other better. She shared about her organization, BTR, and her dream that this organization would be the training ground for Black therapists becoming IFS-trained clinicians. She spoke with such exuberance and conviction that I took to the idea immediately, asking how I could be a part of this vision. We both believed that the model could help heal Black people who have experienced a multitude of traumas. From that point, I worked with Deran and BTR in pursuing the goal of educating Black therapists about IFS and encouraging them to pursue training in the model.

BTR is a non-profit organization of Black professionals, mostly therapists, committed to decreasing stigma and barriers to psychological and social well-being among people of African descent and other vulnerable populations. These goals are accomplished through therapist support, training, and community outreach. BTR is a place for mentorship, networking, and professional development (see www.blacktherapistsrock.com).

DOI: 10.4324/9781003044864-6

After working with Deran for about a year, she approached me to become the IFS consultant to the BTR community. I eagerly accepted. My responsibilities include providing individual and group consultation, business consultation, private practice development, training, and coordination for IFS-I's Organizational Training Program (OTP). This program provides IFS Level 1 training at a reduced rate to clinicians and agencies that work with historically marginalized communities. The relationship between BTR and IFS-I's OTP has been the catalyst for increased interest and involvement of Black therapists in IFS trainings.

A major part of my role as the IFS Consultant to BTR is to identity and prepare members who are interested in taking the IFS Level 1 training. This includes reviewing applications for potential training participants and program assistants and making the appropriate selections. A program assistant (PA) is a member of the training staff who has completed at least a Level 1 training. Ultimately, my goal is to become the IFS lead trainer for the BTR trainings. To that end, I have served as both a PA and assistant trainer for the BTR-IFS training. This training is unique in that it is comprised mostly of Black clinicians, as much as two-thirds to three-quarters. Often clinicians that represent other BIPOC populations (Black, Indigenous, and People Of Color) choose to attend this training also. Typically, the balance of the training is White people. With such a rich group of diverse professionals, this training centers on issues such as systemic racism, social justice, and adaptation of the IFS model to be more inclusive of the needs of the BIPOC community. This collaboration between BTR and IFS-I has multiple benefits. First, it increases the number of Black therapists trained in IFS. This model is desperately needed in their communities to treat the significant traumas experienced by Black people. Second, it allows the participants to interact with a greater number of Black therapists and build new networks, make professional relationships, and create support as they apply the model to their communities. Third, it allows the unique experiences of Black clinicians and the populations they serve to be known and appreciated within the IFS community. With the ongoing training of Black clinicians and encouragement for them to serve as program assistants and assistant trainers, the overall goal is to create an all-Black BTR-IFS leadership training team.

Making Training Accessible

Another goal of BTR is to make the IFS training highly accessible and to educate potential participants about the model in a general sense before making a commitment to the training. In preparation for the 2020 Level 1 training, BTR organized an IFS Question and Answer session for the first time. Although the training is offered at a discount, it is still a substantial amount to pay and requires significant time away from work. Potential training participants want to know what they will receive for their investment. The Q&A

gives the community an opportunity to ask questions about the training and learn how IFS will benefit their practice and professional development. The 2020 Q&A was a success with over 40 mental health professionals in attendance. The attendees left the Q&A equipped with valuable IFS information to assist them in their decision to attend the training. Many decided to sign up for the Level 1 training.

In addition to the Q&A session, I put together for BTR a three-hour training entitled, "Introduction to IFS: What to Know Before Taking Level 1." This training served as an introduction to IFS for participants who are not Level 1 trained and as a refresher course for those who are Level 1 trained and interested in being on the training staff as program assistants. (PAs assist the trainers by supporting participants in the learning objectives of the training and skill building through practice.) The course included background information about the development of IFS therapy, an introduction to parts and Self-energy, foundational knowledge of beginning an IFS session using the 6 Fs (Find, Focus, Flesh Out, Feel toward, beFriend, Fears), and two experiential exercises commonly used in IFS to give the participants a felt sense of parts and Self-energy. From this Introduction to IFS, participants were offered the opportunity to join a consultation group. The 2020 consultation group was led by me and Chris Burris, who is a senior lead trainer for IFS-I and a therapist and consultant. This first Introduction to IFS training for BTR was attended by over 25 people, and ten went on to participate in the consultation group. It is our intention to make the Q&A session, the Introduction to IFS, and the consultation group available each time a BTR-IFS training is held. See Figure 6.1 for a visual representation, which includes these steps in the process of graduating.

BTR Consultation Group

The consultation group is comprised of Level 1 trained clinicians and those yet to be trained. The group serves two purposes: (1) to assist members in developing skills to improve interactions with their clients, and (2) to prepare members for PA positions to assist IFS Level 1 participants. The consultation group provides prospective PAs with insight into their role as PAs and a deepening of their knowledge about the model. This is accomplished by ascertaining their growing edge in the model to better enable them to assist their clients and the participants of the training. This five-week consultation process breaks out as follows:

Session 1 – Teaching on Unblending

Unblending is a foundational skill in working with clients. In order for a client to get to know a part, the client must be able to be with the part and not be the part. This involves separating from the part's feelings, beliefs, and behaviors and moving into the witness position. After the teaching on

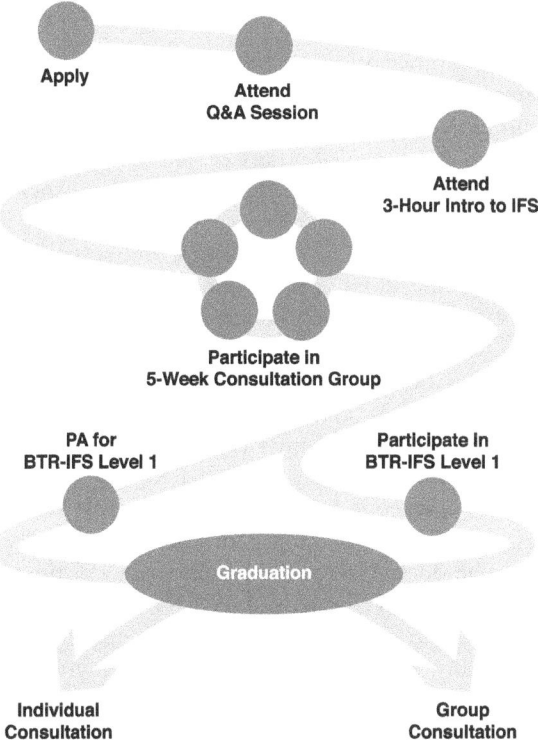

Figure 6.1 From Application to Graduation

unblending, group members are sent into practice triads made up of a client, therapist, and observer to practice the skill of unblending.

Session 2 – Teaching on the Critic

The critic is a part most people possess. It criticizes our thoughts, behaviors, beliefs, and perceptions and makes us feel bad about ourselves. However, like all parts, the critic is attempting to protect. The teaching covers how the critic shows up, its attempts to protect, how it interacts with other parts in the system, and how to work with the critic.

Session 3 – Mapping

Mapping is a method used to externalize the parts of a client's system. Several mapping techniques are covered. The group members are taken through a mapping exercise of their parts. The mapping session ends with an explanation of when to use mapping and the benefits of externalizing parts, and the consultant provides examples of how they use mapping with their clients.

Session 4 – Identity

The consultation conversation on identity focuses on code-switching: "code-switching involves adjusting one's style of speech, appearance, behavior, and expression in ways that will optimize the comfort of others in exchange for fair treatment, quality service, and employment opportunities" (McCluney et al., 2019). Members of the group share their experiences of having to downplay or denounce aspects of themselves to receive quality treatment, acknowledgment, job promotions, and acceptance in the workplace. Members of the 2020 consultation group discussed the effort and stress involved in constantly having to assess White spaces to determine how they should present themselves to increase fair treatment. Some in the group spoke of this behavior as a skill. The ability to move in different worlds and fit in is a type of bilingualism – the ability to communicate verbally and behaviorally in a manner conducive to the environment. After many examples of code-switching were shared, the conversation changed to: What is the cost of code-switching? A similar message was echoed by many in the group. Code-switching comes at a cost of fully being oneself. The need to not be oneself to receive acceptance sends the message that we are somehow unacceptable or flawed. Yet code-switching is a skill that helps those who can do it get their needs met, while those who cannot are excluded from many arenas. One member of our group shared about a company that wanted to hire Black employees but found that those who could code-switch were a better fit in the company culture than those who could not. The conversation ended with the realization that in today's climate of systemic racism, injustice, and police brutality, code-switching is a necessary tool to increase safety and inclusion while hopefully decreasing the likelihood of unjust treatment.

Bringing together Black clinicians and creating an environment of safety allows space for this type of deep and rich exchange. It illuminates the reality of common experiences and creates an opportunity to develop ways to mitigate the impact of these experiences. Just as these clinicians are faced with the impact of code-switching, so are their clients. Therefore, understanding the significance and impact of code-switching will help clinicians assist clients who are faced with it.

Session 5 – Open Forum for Questions

For the open forum session, the group is divided into those who want to PA and those who are participants. For the 2020 consultation group, there were five members in each of the two groups. The PA group presents information related to the PA role, such as guidelines for coaching practice groups and leading reflection groups, while the participant group covers topics such as using IFS with suicidal clients, couples, legacy burdens, or any other topic of interest to the group.

Moving forward, the path to funnel members of the BTR community into the IFS Level 1 training will include a Q&A session to introduce the IFS training and its benefits, followed by the Introduction to IFS, which will present foundational information about IFS and basic concepts as well as an opportunity to join a consultation group to learn more about IFS, enhance skills, and prepare for the PA role. After taking the Level 1 training, participants will be invited to a consultation group to deepen their knowledge and skills within the model (see Figure 6.1).

BTR Individual Consultation

The individual consultation processes that I offer consultees naturally divides into three broad categories (see Figure 6.2): (1) I field questions related to the application of the IFS model, (2) we engage in role-play to model and

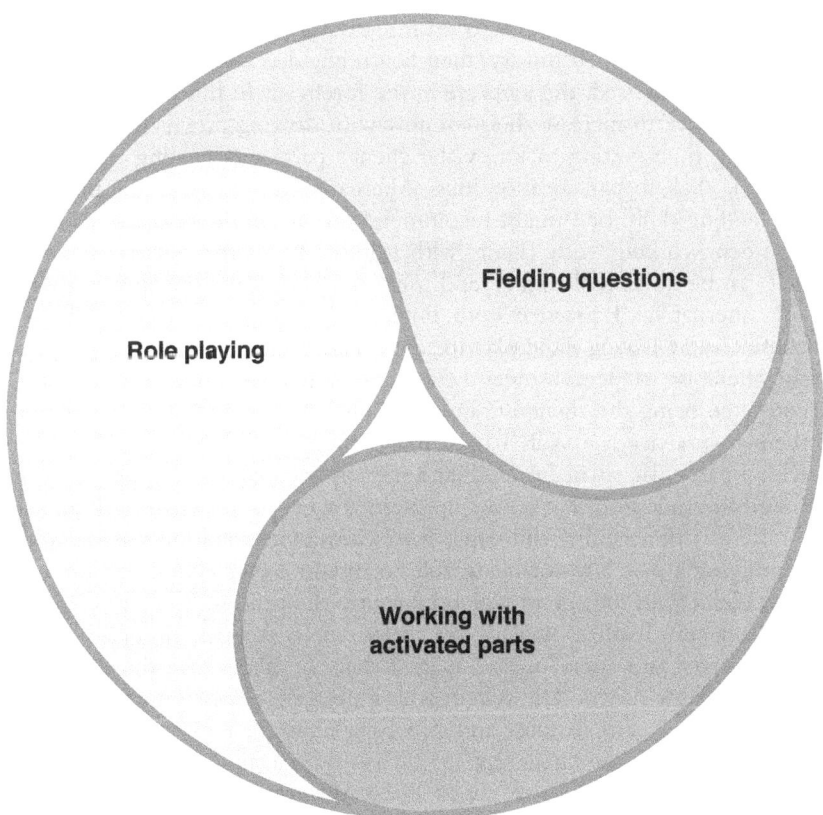

Figure 6.2 The Three Aspects of BTR-IFS Individual Consultation

learn skills to work with challenging clients, and (3) I work with parts of my consultees that get activated when they work with their clients. Although the populations my consultees work with are diverse, they tend to work with clients with significant trauma histories, members of marginalized groups like people of color, members of the LGBTQIA community, and impoverished populations in general. Consultees express the challenges they experience in applying the model to their client work, such as struggling to help the client access Self-energy or ineffectively managing multiple parts surfacing together.

Typical questions include concerns about whether the client has access to Self-energy. This varies from suspecting the client has no Self-energy, minimal Self-energy, or limited ability to maintain Self-energy. The model asserts, "We are all born with a Self. It does not develop through stages or borrow strength and wisdom from the therapist, and it cannot be damaged" (Schwartz & Sweezy, 2020, p. 43). Therefore, my consultees' concerns about the absence of Self in their clients is unfounded. Certainly, there are times when clients have limited or varying access to Self. My approach when these issues come up is to reassure my consultee that their clients have a Self and due to their history, their Self is blended with parts. Instead of the Self being expressed, the parts are in the forefront. In this case, I work with the consultee to increase their comfort with slowing down the process and spending time getting to know the client's parts and assisting the client in building Self-to-part relationships. Alternatively, we focus on improving unblending skills, or I might recommend the use of direct access.

When working with clients with significant trauma histories, accessing Self can be quite challenging, and using the Self of the therapist is a workable alternative. I practice both unblending and direct access skills with consultees by having them play the role of their client, and I take the role of the therapist to demonstrate these skills. Then we trade roles, with the consultee being the therapist, and I act out the role of the client, allowing them to practice the skills I have just demonstrated. This practice is done with a particular client in mind, and the experiential learning broadens out.

Another question that comes up often is what to do when multiple parts interfere with accessing the target part? Consultees bring up the struggle of identifying a part but not being able to sustain a connection because other parts blend with the client, which interrupts the process. Some typical client parts that are hard to manage are intellectuals, skeptics, dissociative parts, fearful parts, and angry ones. I suggest that consultees take this as an indication to slow down. The system is in a protective stance for good reason. Simply asking parts to relax and step back may not move the process forward. Often my consultees have tried that to no avail. My recommendation here is to take the time to get to know the parts that keep showing up. These parts need to be seen and understood before they will allow access to the target part. The use of the 6 Fs is quite useful with these parts, especially the step of befriending, as this increases the part's trust in the Self. Yes, it slows down the process initially, but going slow often helps move the process forward at a quicker rate than trying to unblend and getting stalled over and over again. If this means getting to know multiple parts that interfere with getting to know the target part, I advise taking the time to do so, as these parts took on their protective roles for good reason and will not give up their roles without first being known and building trust with the Self of the client or the therapist.

Working with a Client Suspected of DID

Most of my consultees work with clients with severe and significant trauma histories, and occasionally there is concern that a client has dissociative identity disorder (DID). The DSM-5 defines DID as a "disruption of identity characterized by two or more distinct personality states, which may be described in some cultures as an experience of possession" (American Psychiatric Association, 2013, p. 155). In my experience, the suspicion of this diagnosis is troubling to consultees. They question their ability to treat their client if this is or might be the diagnosis.

I had a consultee who had a part that believed she could not effectively help a client she suspected had DID. This part's disbelief in the therapist's ability caused therapy to stall. I asked her if she would like to get to know this part better. She agreed. The following is an excerpt from our work together.

I asked, "Where do you notice this part in or around your body?"

"In my head, like a nagging pain," she answered.

"Focus on the part and see what you notice."

"It's expanding, filling my head. The pain is more intense."

"Can you be with the pain, or does it need to lessen?"

"No, it's okay."

"Good. What else do you notice."

"The part is telling me to stop before I cause harm. It is afraid that I will hurt my client in some way. It believes I don't know enough to help someone with DID."

"Where did this part get that belief?"

"It says I haven't been trained in DID."

"How do you feel toward this part?"

"I want to know why it thinks I can't handle my client."

I ask the consultee to extend her curiosity to the part and see how it responds. When she does, she notices that her head hurts less. I instruct her to ask the part what it wants her to know.

"The part responds, 'DID clients are scary, dangerous, and unpredictable. You never know what will happen with them'."

"What else does the part want you to know?"

"It says I need to stick to what is safe and what I know how to do."

"Ask the part what its role is."

The consultee answers, "It says its role is to keep me safe from what is scary or dangerous."

"Ask the part how it accomplishes its role."

"The part says it keeps me uncertain when things are unsafe. It makes me fear moving forward, and it makes me question myself and my abilities."

"Ask the part how long it has been doing its role."

"Since I was three," the consultee reports. She continues, saying, "The part is showing me a flash of my chaotic childhood. I always felt unsafe and scared because of my parents' constant fighting."

"Ask the part, how old it thinks you are."

"The part believes I'm five years old."

I tell her to update the part by showing or telling it what has happened in her life since she was five. After the updating, the part responds with surprise and admiration for what she has overcome and accomplished in her life.

"Ask the part what it is afraid will happen if it allows you to work with the client."

"The part is afraid I will get hurt, and its job is to make sure I'm not hurt."

With further questioning, we discovered that this part protects a vulnerable, young part that has been hurt and is very fearful. In later sessions we were able to unburden the consultee's exile. While working with the consultee's parts over several sessions, she was able to continue working with the client using the IFS model. The more we worked with her parts, the more confident she became in her work with her client.

Therapist Self-Awareness

As an IFS therapist, it is imperative that consultees have a sense of self-awareness. Self-awareness is defined as "momentary recognition of and attention to their immediate thoughts, emotions, physiological responses, and behaviors during a therapy session" (Williams & Fauth, 2005, p. 68). The therapist/consultee has two tasks when working with their clients. They are being a parts detector for the client while also being attentive to their own parts activated during the session. It is important that the consultee is aware when their own parts get activated in order to engage unblending techniques. If not, the session becomes a part-to-part interaction instead of an interaction involving the therapist's Self.

Mojta, Falconier, and Huebner (2014) found that IFS helped build therapist self-awareness, which benefited the therapeutic relationship by increasing awareness of therapists' personal agendas, modeling internal awareness to clients, and increasing awareness of clients' internal processes. Self-awareness is an important part of the consultation process. Consultees are encouraged to track their emotions, thoughts, perceptions, also known as their parts, and bring what they discover to their consultation to explore in depth. The exploration includes gaining understanding of why parts are showing up, what they need, and how to work with parts to increase therapist Self-energy.

Hopelessness Legacy Burden

Sinko (2017) provides a protocol for unburdening legacy burdens, which she defines as "the intergenerational transmission of constraining, negative feelings and beliefs" (p. 164). Many of my consultees and clients of color have some understanding of ancestors, generational curses, and generational blessing or gifts, which are the same as legacy burdens and gifts. They also tend to honor and have respect for elders and ancestors. I find that adapting Sinko's protocol for the BIPOC population to incorporate key concepts of "ancestral reverence" (Foor, 2017, p. 81) creates a powerful experience for the client and deepens both the unburdening and the connection with ancestors.

My legacy unburdening practice differs in the unburdening and invitation steps. In the usual protocol, the client's part determines how the ancestor releases the burden and then directs them to do so. Similarly, in the invitation step we ask the client's part what qualities they would like to invite into their system, and they instruct the ancestor at the end of the line to take those qualities in and pass them forward. Instead of directing the client's part to guide the unburdening and invitation, I invite the ancestors to guide both processes. These changes reflect two important aspects of ancestral reverence. The first is that when relating with ancestors "a witness state" of "look but don't touch" is maintained (Foor, 2017, p. 81). Where possible, when interacting with ancestors our role is to witness and avoid the impulse to help or intervene. The second aspect involves avoiding "the hubris of assuming that our help is invited or that we understand what actually constitutes help in any given situation" (Foor, 2017, p. 82). We remain aware that we don't know what we don't know, and we trust that the ancestors do know what help is needed. The vignette that follows illustrates one way to invite this active involvement of the ancestors.

Through self-awareness and tracking of her parts, a consultee named Lynette noticed a hopeless part in relation to a female client with a significant trauma history. Lynette had worked with the client for 14 months when she brought her concerns to one of our sessions. She explained that the client had experienced years of sexual exploitation as a child while in the care of a babysitter. The consultee reported that after over a year of working with the client, she had not unburdened any exiles. Whenever they got close to an exile, protectors would undermine the process. Lynette described the client as having little Self-energy and explained that she often uses direct access. She states that the client's parts respond to her Self-energy but don't trust the client. When the client has any amount of Self-energy, she gets overwhelmed by the intensity of her parts and will ask Lynette to talk directly to them. Lynette is a trauma specialist in private practice, and both she and the client are Black. She states that she feels hopeless with clients who she perceives as having less Self-energy or those with whom she has worked for a long time with little improvement. She admits that with these clients she feels ineffective and questions her abilities as a therapist. "I always feel hopeless when things get hard," Lynette admits through tears. I am curious. I wonder if some of her hopelessness is connected to a legacy burden since she states she "always" feels hopeless when things get hard. I ask Lynette if her hopelessness feels like a legacy burden; if any amount of the hopelessness feels like it doesn't belong to her. She sits pensively for a moment and answers, "My mother was hopeless and sad a lot of the time, especially when she felt life wasn't working out for her. So, yes this could be legacy too."

"Lynette, would you like to release the portion of the hopelessness that does not belong to you?"

"Yes."

"Answer this next question without trying to figure it out. Whatever comes to mind, go with it. What percentage of the hopelessness seems to not be yours?"

"About 70 percent."

"Is there any reason you or any of your parts need to hold onto this burden?"

"No."

"Okay. I'd like you to invite the Self of your mother and any other ancestors you inherited this burden from. This includes both known and unknown ancestors who carry the burden of hopelessness."

Lynette sits quietly then slightly nods her head and says, "I'm remembering a time I walked into the kitchen and saw my mother sitting at the table looking at papers in a small box. She's crying and looks distraught. I watch until she puts the lid on the box and places it on top of the refrigerator. After she leaves, I go and look in the box. It is filled with bills, many say 'Past Due' on them."

(Lynette refers to a younger part who took on the burden of hopelessness through Lynette's personal experience. This part is unburdened later.)

"How do you feel toward your mother?"

"I feel compassion for her. I know she felt hopeless. I think this was after she and my father broke up."

"What about your other ancestors, how do you feel toward them?"

"The same. I have compassion for them too."

"Take the hopelessness you inherited from your mother out of your body and pass it back to her."

After Lynette does this, I ask her to have her mother take the burden from her body and pass it to the ancestor she inherited it from. The process is continued with each ancestor until the end of the line is reached.

This is the point where my protocol diverges. Instead of having the client's part identify how to release the burden, the ancestor determines how the burden is released. The ancestor also identifies the positive qualities to invite into the ancestral line. Allowing the ancestor to choose in what way to release the burden and which positive qualities to invite makes sense considering we are dealing with the portion of the burden that didn't belong to the client. It also honors the ancestor's knowing of the best way to heal the ancestral line.

When the last ancestor is reached, I say, "Ask the ancestor to release the legacy burden how they see fit. When that process is complete let me know."

I sit quietly holding Self-energy for several minutes during this process.

"It's complete."

"Now ask the ancestor what positive qualities they might want to invite into the line."

"The ancestor invites confidence, capability, smarts, trust, and a knowing that life will work out."

"Ask the ancestor how they would like to share these wonderful qualities with the ancestral line and let me know when that process is complete."

When the process is complete, Lynette nods. I invite her to see how her parts and ancestors are doing and to check if anything else is needed by anyone. She answers, "Everything is good."

"Invite any parts who need to see the change and be updated to come forth."

"My remaining hopeless part likes the change and wants to change too."

"Let the part know that we will work with it in a future session … Take the time to thank your parts and ancestors for the work they did today."

At the end of the session the consultee reports feeling lighter and more expansive. In subsequent sessions with her client, she finds herself feeling more confident and less bothered by the client's level of Self-energy. She notices that the client requests direct access less and maintains Self-energy slightly longer.

Adaptations to the Model

My consultees and the clients they serve tend to be members of the BIPOC population. I have found that applying the IFS model requires adjustments to meet the needs of this population. I use these changes when working with my consultees and encourage them to utilize them with their clients if they seem beneficial. The areas that are different with BIPOC clients/consultees include storytelling, externalizing parts, extended befriending, not asking parts to step back, and listening for and unburdening legacy burdens (see Table 6.1).

The IFS model encourages a relationship between parts and the Self. However, while working with a target part, another part may intervene. In order to focus on the target part, the intervening part will be asked to relax or step aside to allow the target part to continue. I have found that when

Table 6.1 Five Key Adaptations When Working with Clients from the BIPOC Population

Welcoming the Storyteller	**Externalizing**
Welcome and befriend the Storyteller part – it can provide missing information, historical details, or a unique perspective.	Assist clients to represent inner parts in the outside world using parts mapping, IFS parts cards and miniatures before interviewing them as usual.
Extended befriending	
Slow down the befriending process to ensure the part feels known by Self and has experienced Self-energy. There may be a lack of trust in Self and over-reliance on parts who have had to manage historical threats.	
Getting to know parts rather than asking them to step back	**Listen for and unburden legacy burdens**
Spending time with parts as they arise, even if they are not the target part, allows the client to learn about their system and increases trust and connection internally.	Get curious about behaviors, emotions, mental health issues, and repeated patterns as possibly being tied to a legacy burden. Unburdening these first opens up more space inside, allowing greater access to Self in both client and consultee.

the intervening part is a storytelling part, it may be necessary to invite this part to share its story. With the BIPOC population, I see the existence of this part regularly. When attempts are made to have this part step back in this population, it tends to resist. It wants to share its stories. I find that engaging the Storyteller builds trust within the system of which it is part. Sometimes this part has information not accessible to the target part, or it has a new and different perspective on the situation being discussed. This is an example of going slow to go far. By not rushing to get to know the target part and spending some time with the Storyteller (going slow), the process often goes farther and sometimes faster because time is spent listening to and building relationship with the Storyteller. In cases where the Storyteller is ignored or asked to step back, it may cause upset within the system by refusing to step aside and shutting down access to the target part. It is advisable when this part presents to spend time building a Self-to-part relationship and listening to what the part has to offer. All of which are reason enough to take the time to get to know this part.

Some of my consultees have shared their difficulty in helping clients who are members of the BIPOC population connect with and/or identify parts. This may partially be attributed to the fact that many of their clients have also experienced significant trauma, including racial trauma. In these cases, externalizing parts is a helpful tool. Externalizing parts includes using techniques to assist the client in relocating parts from inside of them to outside. I recommend the use of the following tools to facilitate this process: mapping, the use of miniatures, and IFS parts cards.

These tools are used by having the client go inside and locate a part. The part may present as an emotion, physical sensation, image, sound, or words. Once the client has a sense of the part, the client is instructed to draw it (if mapping is used) or select a miniature or IFS parts card that most closely represents the part. Once the part has been externalized, questions can be posed to the part to get to know it better. Questions include:

1   What does the part want you to know about itself?
2   How do you feel toward the part?
3   What might the part need from you?

After getting to know a part by externalizing it, a client may be better able to remain unblended as they work through the 6 Fs and healing steps.

Another process that needs to be adjusted for the BIPOC population is befriending. Befriending is one of the 6 Fs in the relationship-building process of the IFS model. Befriending "involves learning about the target part and developing a friendly relationship. This builds relationship internally (Self to part) and externally (part to therapist)" (Anderson et al., 2017, p. 38). Befriending establishes trust between the therapist and the part as the therapist facilitates the relationship between the Self of the client and the part. This population can have a distrust of Self. This may be due to parts needing to come to the fore to protect the system from outside threats in the past. The lack of trust and lack of reliance on the Self is why it is advisable to extend the befriending process. The process can be extended by spending more time with the target part building the Self-to-part relationship. Slowing down the process is important at this point, ensuring that the part feels known by the Self and has an experience of Self-energy before moving forward.

Another adjustment of standard procedure when working with the BIPOC population is not asking parts to step back when they show up while working with a target part. Taking time to allow the client to learn about their system by spending time with parts as they show up increases trust and connection, which improves the ease of working within the system as the process evolves. These parts usually have good information to impart, even if they are motivated by their fear of allowing engagement with the target part. Therefore, engage the parts that interrupt the process. Ask them what they have to offer. The exchange may result in the part becoming the new target part, or the process may resume with the original part. Either way, spending time with parts as they present themselves helps the client learn their system and build relationship with the parts involved. These parts usually have a good reason to protect the target part or hinder access to it and progress through the steps of healing.

An awareness of legacy burdens is particularly important to the therapeutic process with this population. I emphasize the importance of listening for legacy burdens with my consultees. Members of the BIPOC population often carry legacy burdens, and developing the skills for identifying and unburdening them is imperative for professionals who work with this population. Legacy burdens are easier to unburden than personal burdens because they do not belong to the person – they were inherited or passed down. If the legacy burden is unburdened first, it will open more space in the system allowing greater access to Self. The increased access to Self-energy will help facilitate the work of healing the client's personal burdens.

I challenge my consultees to get curious about their own and their clients' behaviors, emotions, mental health issues, and repeated patterns as possibly being tied to a legacy burden. For Black clients, legacy burdens may be connected to historical events, like slavery or Jim Crow laws and brutality. Current events may also fuel legacy burdens, like the disproportionate incarceration of Black men, absent Black fathers, and police brutality. Even mental health issues, such as depression and anxiety, emotional states of hopelessness, feeling not good enough, or shame, may indicate the presence of a legacy burden. I am aware of cases with consultees and in my own practice when personal unburdening occurs first and the mental health issue resurfaces. This may be a point to inquire about the presence of a legacy burden. Sometimes the issue reappears because the legacy burden has not been addressed.

Conclusion

We teach best what we most need to learn (Bach, 1998).

I have experienced my position as the IFS Consultant to BTR as part calling, part professional development, and part teacher. My role is part calling because I knew instantly as I sat in my Level 1 training that the IFS model of therapy was exactly what I and other Black professionals need to take our practices to the next level and enable us to make a greater impact with our clients. I felt drawn to having an active role in training therapists to help heal our communities. Finding myself in the same training as Deran Young was not an accident. We were meant to meet and forge a connection to work together in bringing IFS to the community of Black mental health professionals in America. My desire to spread the message of IFS through the community motivated me to take Levels 2 and 3 and become certified. I was called to learn as much as I possibly could about the model. My experience has been part professional development in that I learn a wealth of information from my consultees. Hearing about their cases and the original ways in which they interact with their clients makes me a better clinician and consultant. I am privy to various creative ways to use the model with different populations in a variety of settings. I am also tasked with finding answers to some difficult questions, which keeps me learning as much as I can. Lastly, my role is part teacher. I believe that I am teaching what I most need to learn. My consultees come to me with challenging cases, questions, and blocks created by their own parts. They are highly committed to their clients and want to learn as much as possible to improve their skills. Teaching this model to others sharpens my skill set, which increases the value of my consultation services to the BTR community.

References

American Psychiatric Association. (2013). *Diagnostic and statistical manual of mental disorders, fifth edition* (DSM-5). American Psychiatric Publishing.

Anderson, F., Sweezy, M., & Schwartz, R. C. (2017). *Internal Family Systems, skills training manual: Trauma-informed treatment for anxiety, depression, PTSD & substance abuse.* PESI.

Bach, R. (1998). *Illusions: The adventures of a reluctant messiah.* Arrow Books.

Foor, D. (2017). *Ancestral medicine: Rituals for personal and family healing.* Bear and Company.

McCluney, C. L., Robotham, K., Lee, S., Smith, R., & Durkee, M. (2019, November 15). The costs of code-switching. *Harvard Business Review.* https://hbr.org/2019/11/the-costs-of-codeswitching.

Mojta, C., Falconier, M. K., & Huebner, A. J. (2014, December 23). Fostering self-awareness in novice therapists using Internal Family Systems therapy. *The American Journal of Family Therapy, 42*(1), 67–78. doi:10.1080/01926187.2013.772870.

Schwartz, R. C, & Sweezy, M. (2020). *Internal Family Systems therapy* (2nd ed.). The Guilford Press.

Sinko, A. L. (2017) Legacy Burdens. In M. Sweezy & E. L. Ziskind (Eds.), *Innovations and elaborations in Internal Family Systems therapy* (pp. 164–178). Routledge.

Williams, E. N., & Fauth, J. (2005). A psychotherapy process study of therapist in session self-awareness. *Psychotherapy Research, 15*(4), 374–381. doi:10.1080/10503300500091355.

7 Trusting Self to Heal

Removing Constraints to Therapists' Self-Energy Transforms Their Treatment of Eating Disordered Clients

Jeanne Catanzaro

Introduction

I commonly encounter clinicians who say things like "I don't work with eating issues." Their discomfort is obvious in comments like "I'm not good at that" and "How can I help someone else if I can't help myself?" The reality is we all "work with" eating issues to some extent. We all have burdens related to food and our bodies, even if we don't experience them as problematic or extreme. Clinicians who become aware of the fears and biases they hold about food and bodies will be more effective at helping clients heal. At a minimum, they will be more Self-led and less likely to do harm to clients by avoiding or not noticing parts of the client that are in pain. Getting to know their parts who are fearful or overwhelmed by the more extreme manifestations of eating issues helps clinicians stay Self-led to better negotiate the complex and often extreme behaviors associated with these disorders.

The ubiquity of eating disorders and disordered eating in Western culture underscores the need for more clinicians who can identify and treat these conditions. In this chapter, I discuss how I use the Internal Family Systems (IFS) model in consultation to help clinicians develop a sense of competence in understanding and working with protectors who focus on food and the body to manage feelings and to cope with various traumatic experiences. Using case vignettes from my clinical practice, I describe the challenges involved in working with clinicians who vary in terms of their professional backgrounds, their experience with eating issues, and their knowledge of and proficiency with the IFS model. I address common challenges that arise in my work with IFS trained clinicians, such as when the clinician's grasp of IFS remains largely intellectual or when parts of the clinician interfere with the treatment. Throughout this chapter I illustrate how I work with the parts of the clinician and myself that get activated by each other, the client, the family system, and/or the larger culture. I describe the frustration associated with particularly extreme or entrenched systems and how to negotiate these stuck points. Finally, I provide examples of cases where clinicians experience deep satisfaction from observing the

DOI: 10.4324/9781003044864-7

transformation that results when they successfully work with their own parts and avoid the power struggles so common to typical approaches to eating disorder treatment.

It All Began with Eating Disorders

The IFS model grew out of Richard Schwartz's work with eating disordered clients. This is important to note, since eating disorders and disordered eating are so often viewed as destructive, irrational conditions. At an impasse in his treatment with his clients, Dick stopped trying to fix them and instead got curious about their experiences and what kept them stuck in painful patterns of thinking, feeling, and behaving. He discovered that these symptoms emanated from different parts of the internal system who adopted them to cope with all kinds of difficulties. While they could seem extreme, rigid, or chaotic, they made sense given the client's history. In addition to these parts, clients also described having a deeper healing energy, a core wisdom IFS refers to as the Self, which is present in even the most traumatized individual.

These revelations changed the way IFS therapists treat eating disorders and eating issues of all kinds. Instead of trying to manage or eliminate the eating-related thoughts and behaviors, techniques that typically result in power struggles or temporary compliance, IFS clinicians pay attention to them to understand their intended purpose. Trusting that within each client is a Self who knows how to heal the parts, they shift from trying to "do something" about the thoughts and behaviors to getting curious about them, which engenders the client's own respect for and curiosity about them. In other words, IFS clinicians create the conditions for clients to get into Self and extend Self-energy to the parts who focus on food and the body, providing, at last, a way to shift out of habitual and self-limiting modes of protection. IFS consultation aims to do the same for the consulting clinician.

Creating the Conditions for Self-Led Consultation

Getting and staying curious about behaviors that are often frustrating and frightening is challenging. Eating disorders and disordered eating are complicated issues that can have serious physical and emotional consequences and typically involve interacting with others (e.g., family, friends, doctors) who have strong feelings about what should be happening in the treatment. IFS consultation for disordered eating and eating disorders helps clinicians get to know and work with the parts of themselves that arise as they negotiate these difficulties.

Over the last five years, I have been researching the different ways legacy burdens of all kinds impact how people relate to food and their bodies. I've learned a great deal from those who have devoted themselves to healing the social inequity and stigma that keep people stuck in painful relationships with food and their bodies (Be Nourished, n.d.; Cox, 2020; Harrison, 2019; Piran, 2017; Taylor, 2018). From this immersion, I came to new awareness about what the clinical setting has been historically willing and unwilling to address. First and foremost, I learned that none of us is exempt from the cultural waters in which we swim, filled as all cultures are with ideals of beauty and experiences of shame. This makes it imperative that we clinicians explore our own burdens and investigate their impact on what we see and how we respond to the different burdens of our clients.

In the initial session I explore the consultee's reasons for consultation and what they are hoping to get from our work together. I ask them about their prior clinical training and their experience with eating disorders and disordered eating. Finally, I ask the consultee about their level of training in and comfort with the IFS model. My initial consultation with Melissa and Robin illustrates the way I set the stage for our consulting relationship. Social workers in their mid-30s, they contacted me after completing their Level 1 IFS training. Like many IFS therapists who specialize in the treatment of eating disorders, they reported a lack of local IFS resources (consultants, colleagues, dietitians, treatment programs) on which they could rely for guidance and help with referrals as well as nutritional and medical backup. Both women related that the dearth of support was the primary reason they sought consultation and also why they opted to meet together rather than individually.

As I explored their expectations for consultation, I made a suggestion, "While you sought supervision for help with clients' eating disorders, I propose that this be a laboratory of sorts for increasing your ability to be skillful parts detectors for all kinds of burdens related to food and bodies, if that feels comfortable to you. I will invite each of you to reflect on your own experiences as we discuss these cases. I will also be tracking the parts that come up within my system, asking them to give me space so I can be curious and speaking for them when I feel like it might be helpful to share as they arise in response to the clinical material."

Melissa responded by saying, "For me I'm certainly open to looking at my own parts and the ones that get activated in session. I have my own history of eating issues and a period of time where I probably would have been considered eating disordered."

Robin nodded and said, "I've never had significant issues about eating or my body, aside from minor ups and downs in terms of how I feel about myself, but my sister was bullied for being fat when we were kids, and as an adult she's still concerned about it, so I know parts of me have some fallout from that."

Both women agreed to explore the parts that were getting activated in their sessions and in our consultation group. I described the parameters for our discussions as a group: "Understanding that this is not therapy, there are times when it might be useful for one or both of you to explore more fully the parts that come up, to see what they're responding to, what they're protecting, and to see if we can help you unblend more. I'll always check with you to see if it feels comfortable for both of you to do this, the one who's doing the work and the one who's observing."

With its emphasis on creating a safe space where "all parts are welcome," IFS consultation can be very helpful in reducing the isolation, frustration, and overwhelm common to many who work with eating- and body-related issues. This safety is crucial to help clinicians unblend from the parts that get triggered by frightening physical symptoms; suicidality and other extreme firefighters; inadequate financial, medical, and nutritional support; and polarized relationships with family members and other providers. The following vignettes illustrate some of the most common reasons people seek consultation and how these issues can be negotiated to increase the Self-energy available to help our clients get curious about and heal their own systems.

Patty: The Lure of the Familiar

Clinicians who come for consultation vary widely in terms of their educational/professional backgrounds, their IFS training, and their comfort with the IFS model. It takes time to assimilate the teachings of the model, much like it takes time to learn a new language. Clinicians with prior experience with eating disorders can find it challenging to make the shift from talking about parts to helping clients relate to their own parts from Self. For therapists who have been taught that the therapist provides what the client needs to heal (e.g., corrective attachments, information, resources, and skills), this is a very different way of working. In moments where there is a lot of uncertainty or concern for the client, it can be tempting to revert to what is familiar. Patty's work with a client with binge eating disorder is a good example of what this can be like.

I first met Patty when she was finishing her Level 1 training. She felt inspired by learning that eating disorder symptoms are not irrational beliefs and feelings but rather protective parts who have important reasons for doing what they do. This resonated with what she'd observed with her clients, who were often able to articulate how their eating disorders had been helpful to them. Patty was relieved by the prospect of not having to do battle with her clients' eating disorders, which she'd found draining. That said, she found herself feeling thwarted by clients who "resisted" connecting with their parts, preferring instead to report their daily struggles with food and their bodies.

Patty described her work with Diana, a 48-year-old woman who had come to her for help with binge eating disorder and with whom she'd been working for three years: "In the past I would have found myself problem-solving with her about how to handle her evenings, since that's when most of her bingeing happens. I would have had her notice the thoughts coming in towards the end of the workday, the impulses to buy food on the way home. I would have helped her strategize about what she could do instead of bingeing. And I would have focused on the 'all or nothing,' 'last supper' kind of thinking that inevitably leads to the next binge. Now, instead, I've been working to help her get curious about that moment when she first notices the part that's planning the binge. She realizes how the bingeing part is protecting parts who feel so deprived and overworked. She gets that it's giving her something to look forward to, something to help her unhook and not feel as resentful about how hard she has to work."

Despite this awareness, she said, Diana's binges continue, and critical parts reliably react to them with judgment and new plans to restrict. "In those moments she's not interested in getting to know the exiles, aside from naming them."

I asked Patty if she could check inside and notice any parts who were coming up as she discussed her work with Diana. She said, "I'm feeling stuck and a little frustrated." I asked her if she could listen to the part who felt frustrated and see what it wanted her to know. "It's a little maddening how passive Diana is. She's kind of resigned to the eating disorder, even though she complains about it, especially how much it occupies her time, how much money she spends on food." As Patty focused on her frustrated part, she realized that it was protecting a part who felt responsible for getting Diana to change. I asked Patty if she could ask the responsible part what it feared would happen if it stepped back so she could relate to Diana more from Self. She sighed, "It would be great if I could do that. I hadn't realized how responsible a part of me has been feeling. That part says 'I've been working with her for a long time. If I (the responsible part) were doing a better job, Diana (the client) wouldn't be struggling the way she is.'"

I asked how she felt toward this part of herself. "I feel for it, it works very hard, and I know why. I don't need to go into that now, it's a part I've been getting to know more in my IFS therapy, but I'm starting to realize how often it takes over when I'm with clients, especially ones who have passive or hopeless parts."

After a long pause she added, "I know that the more I let this part of me take over, the less room there is for her [Diana] to step in and take the initiative. But it's really hard to resist the urge to *do* something."

Until she spoke about it in our consultation, Patty hadn't realized how often she'd been blended with her responsible, caretaking manager and how it was affecting her work with Diana. As she described their sessions, I observed how often this part made assumptions about Diana's parts instead of engaging Diana's curiosity about her own experience. Reflecting on this pattern of tracking the sequence of parts and interpreting their motives she said, "That's how I'm used to working, I guess. I think it happens mostly when I'm feeling like we're not getting anywhere because she keeps going from one part to another. A part of me is trying to help her notice how she does this so she'll get it and then we can work with her parts."

Buoyed by our consultation as well as her individual IFS therapy, Patty paid attention to the part who felt responsible for getting Diana unstuck. She reminded her that within Diana was a Self that could be trusted to take care of her own parts, something that would be much more likely to happen if Patty's own part didn't take over in the session. "I had to keep checking in with this part and asking her to be patient, because she kept wanting to interpret or explain. It was hard for her to tolerate Diana's stuckness, if that's a word, until I listened to her (the part) more fully and learned what was making it so hard for her to not be doing something more active. She let me know that it felt really bad to not say something when she had the information that could facilitate things."

As Patty got to know this part further, she realized how young she was and how hard she had tried to protect an exile in her system from feeling out of control by doing something to help the adults around her: "She did this by tracking what was going on, anticipating things, and being the one people could talk to when they were upset." Patty understood better why "not saying or doing anything" felt risky to this part, who had protected parts who were frightened by her parents' dysfunction. "I hadn't realized how active this young protector had been in my sessions. Once I got that, I was able to help her trust that I wasn't that scared girl anymore and that she didn't need to keep coming in to help me or my clients in the way she had been. She knows now that she doesn't even need to be around for the therapy, she can go out and play."

With this shift, Patty noticed how much more effective the therapy was when Diana connected to her parts from her own Self. She (Patty) said, "It was never about ego, but some pre-IFS perceptions I had about what healing means, some ideas about attachment being so important. Now, I really get – and my responsible part gets – that unblending and letting my Self be present to Diana is the 'doing something.'"

Sarah: The Fear of the Unknown

Like Patty, Sarah is also a seasoned clinician with considerable experience working with trauma and eating disorders. She completed her Level 1 training several years prior to contacting me for help with Caroline, a 40-year-old client whose chronic anorexia and depression had worsened after she'd been asked to leave a residential treatment program due to noncompliance. When she related the details of the case, I noticed within myself a part who felt concerned for Sarah. It heard how little support Sarah had to work with a woman whose emotional and physical symptoms and lack of social support were highly concerning. One of the few clinicians who specialized in eating disorders in her region, Sarah was also one of the only IFS therapists. Compounding her clinical concerns was the dearth of intensive outpatient or residential treatment programs in her area and the few physicians and dietitians to whom she felt comfortable referring.

After I listened for a couple of minutes, I paused Sarah and asked her to notice the part who was reporting details of the case. A startled look appeared on her face. "Good question." She took a deep breath and exhaled loudly. "It's like I've got to make sure you know all the details so you can help me." I told her that made sense to me. Faced with the challenges of inadequate treatment resources, poor insurance coverage, and limited psychiatric/medical support, clinicians who work with clients with eating disorders and disordered eating can feel overwhelmed by clients who see them as their only hope – the one person who can fix them. Similarly, consultees frequently can feel that way about me. While it's true that my experience has helped me feel more confident in working with these difficult systems, there are times when I notice a part who believes that someone else with more skill would be better able to help the client with whom I'm working. In that moment, the most helpful thing I can do is get my anxious parts to step back so I can get back into Self.

"While you were describing what's been going on for you, I noticed an anxious part of my own. It shares the concern about how alone it sounds like you've been in your work with Caroline. It's reminding me of times when I've felt quite alone, without an adequate treatment team or referral options."

I told Sarah how I've learned to regard my anxious and resentful parts becoming activated as important warnings that either there's too little support for the case or that I've blended with a part who is attached to healing the client or both. The alliance between parts who hold fear about the client and the ones who try to rescue the client can be quite powerful and can pull clinicians to do things that may not be helpful for themselves or the client. Common examples include parts of the clinician scheduling additional sessions and agreeing to out-of-session contact in the form of emails, texts, and phone calls. While additional support is often called for when working with clients with eating disorders, especially those with complex trauma or those whose parts become more extreme when approaching certain exiles, it is important to consider whether the offer of support comes from a part or from the Self.

Sarah appreciated how parts of me resonated with her experience. "It's helpful to hear you say that. I have many parts who feel stressed, overwhelmed, and alone with this case. When I check in with them about what's the worst thing for them, they say it's two things: the concern about her physical stability and how isolated she is. She's been depressed on and off over the past five years, but this time feels different. She'd attached a lot of hope to the last treatment. The combination of that not working out and her 40th birthday have brought her depression to a new level. Whatever part was able to keep her in denial about a number of things, especially her fertility, just hit its limit with this birthday."

"Do you want to focus on the part or parts who are concerned about her depression?"

"Yes, I think that would be a good idea."

"Okay, great. Would you see if the anxious part has stepped back? If it hasn't, we can ask what it needs from you to relax a little more."

"My sense is that it has stepped back, but let me check."

She closed her eyes for a couple of seconds before opening them, saying, "Yes, it helped to name the anxiety. I think there are parts of me who keep trying to minimize it, push it aside, so I can manage the stress while she waits for a bed to open up at another treatment program. It helps to speak for the anxiety and also to know that you can understand it."

Shifting her attention to Caroline's despair, which spiked when she left the residential treatment program, Sarah recalled, "She was the oldest patient by about 20 years. It was like facing all of the loss at once – her youth, her opportunities for getting married and having her own family. Since then, she's been dominated by her restricting and depressed parts. She's only open to considering another treatment program because she knows I won't continue to work with her on an outpatient basis. She's technically stable at the moment but doesn't have a lot of margin."

I asked Sarah what she noticed as she described Caroline's treatment history and current state. "I have such a hard time getting her to separate from the depressed part, she says 'This is just me.' It never goes anywhere." I asked Sarah whether she'd tried doing direct access with the part. Direct access is a technique that can be helpful when parts of the client don't trust the client's Self enough to relax and unblend. Sarah shook her head. "Not with any good result. But if I'm honest, I'm not sure how well I'm really doing it. I don't do it with any real confidence, and I think I kind of shift into more talking about the depressed part with her."

"Would you be willing to try it here? If you can role-play her, I will do direct access with the depressed part. I can do this in one of two ways: explicitly, by asking her if it would be okay for me to speak directly to her depressed part, or implicitly, where I speak to her as the depressed part. In either case the goal is to connect with the part and listen to its concerns until it trusts that it's safe to separate more from her."

"Oh yeah, that would be great. I think she'd be more open to the implicit direct access." Sarah took a moment and closed her eyes to focus on her experience of Caroline's depressed part and what that part might say. She opened her eyes and said, "This is not a part, it's a fact that I'm too fucked up. Nothing's going to get better. The only thing I'm doing is causing other people pain, the only thing I have is pain. There's nothing you can do, nothing you can say. This is my experience. I'm telling you how I feel."

"I hear you and I want to understand more about you and how you feel, how you see things. You feel like nothing's ever going to get better?" My goal here is to provide the part with the opportunity to feel understood. I do this by repeating what I've heard the part say and opening space for it to share more.

"I'm not feeling that it's ever going to get better, it's true. It's pointless. I've tried everything."

This is a real issue in eating disorder treatment. Clients often go through several therapists or rounds of treatment without much improvement. For clients like Caroline, whose anorexia spans 20 years, the statistics regarding mortality are grim. In moments like these I remind consultees of the importance of the 5 Ps. Presence, perspective, persistence, patience, and playfulness are vital to staying Self-led so we can help clients with entrenched protectors.

"What is it like for you to hold the belief that it's pointless?"

"It's awful. And every time I tell someone that, they tell me I shouldn't feel that way; they list all the reasons why, and then they ask me, 'Are you going to kill yourself? You need to go to a higher level of care.' So, I can't even tell anyone how I'm feeling."

Speaking as Sarah the therapist, I say, "I can understand how that would make you not want to say anything. I realize that there are times in the past when I've done that, when parts of me have blocked me from being curious about you. I'm sorry I've let them take over at times. I've asked them to step back so I can be present right now and hear more about what this is like for you."

Role-playing Sarah's apology is important for several reasons. First, it normalizes the experience of getting blended with parts. Second, it models unblending. Finally, and most importantly, it demonstrates building trust with the eating disordered client, who has likely been managed in the past by parts of the clinicians who want them to either ward off their eating disorder, suicidal or other extreme protectors or try to contract with them so they don't act on their intentions.

Sarah interjected, "As an aside, as you acknowledge how you blended with your parts, I noticed feeling less tension, less bracing in my arms. It feels like you are genuinely curious, not just acting like you are while you're figuring out how to get me, the client, to feel better."

Her comment underscores the importance of getting parts who have an agenda to step back so the clinician's Self-energy comes through.

Getting back into the role-play, "Caroline" continued, "Every time I express these feelings, people just try to shut me down, get me to feel differently."

"I'm getting how hard that's been for you. Do you trust that I am genuinely curious about you right now?"

"Right now, it feels like you are."

(Shifting to explicit direct access) "Okay, great. I also hear how strongly you believe Caroline's tried everything and how pointless it would be for her to hope for anything different. Am I getting this right?"

"Caroline" nodded affirmatively. I continued to explore the depressed part's role in the system. "What are you afraid would happen if you didn't keep reminding her of how pointless it all is?"

"Then she might get her hopes up, only to have them shot down again."

"So, you protect her from being disappointed. What's the worst thing that would happen if she got disappointed again?"

"The worst thing is she would get suicidal."

"A suicidal part would take over? Has that happened before?"

"Yes, the last time she really got her hopes up about treatment, the last time she really thought she would get better, and then she didn't."

"That sounds so painful."

"It was terrible. A suicidal part took over and things got really scary."

"I know that right now you don't believe this is possible, but if we could heal the parts the suicidal part protects, the ones that get so devastated by disappointment, would you have to keep her depressed, or would you rather do something else for her?"

"I'd rather do something else, but I don't think it's possible to heal the ones who feel so devastated."

"I get you don't believe it's possible, but if you give us a chance, we can heal them so they don't get as hurt. Would you be willing to step back a little so we could try that?"

"I'd be open to trying, at least for a little while."

"That's great. That's all we can ask. I appreciate your willingness to take the risk to try something new. Is there anything more you want me to know, or is it okay for me to shift back to 'Caroline'?"

Sarah sighed and said, "Thank you, this feels so helpful. It helps me to experience you do it and to realize how different, how powerful, it feels when you do it from Self. While it doesn't feel easy, it feels like so much less of a battle. It made me realize how parts of me have felt scared of the suicidal part and a little hopeless about getting any traction with the one who blankets everything with depression. I also realize how parts of me have shied away from doing direct access, and I'm seeing how helpful it can be."

Melanie: When What We Don't Know About Our Own System Impedes Another's Healing

Melanie, a clinical psychologist in her mid-50s, contacted me for consultation because she had some questions about a client who had come to her for help with anxiety related to his stressful marriage. After the relationship broke up, Jim needed an outlet for his anxiety and a way to meet other people. He joined a local running club and started a beginner's running program, which would prepare him to run a 5K. An athlete in high school, Jim reconnected with a part of himself he'd missed, one who loved feats of physical exertion and mastery. Soon he was training for a marathon and organized his days and especially weekends around his long runs. For the first time in years, he felt a sense of pride as he completed several half marathons and trained for a full marathon.

Melanie noticed parts of herself feeling somewhat envious of Jim's transformation. Like Jim, she'd been athletic as a young woman and had parts who believed she should be more active now. She was impressed by the improvement in Jim's mood and the other changes he was making in terms of his self-care program. In addition to running, Jim had embarked on an eating program that involved eliminating all flour, sugar, and alcohol; eating meals at set times of the day; and never eating between meals. "He says he loves the clarity, the calm, the fact that he's not thinking about food all day. The voices which used to argue with him about what, when, and how much to eat or bargain with him aren't there anymore." Over the course of three months, Jim had lost a significant amount of weight. His mood was brighter, and he now felt confident enough to start dating again.

Melanie related, "He really needed to lose weight, and he looks great. He's so much less lonely now that he has his running group and the online community for his eating program. The thing is, he's started dating someone in his running club, and his anxiety has gone through the roof. He's started craving alcohol, which is disturbing to him because he's been sober for 15 years."

Melanie described her efforts to help Jim get to know the part who was craving alcohol, to learn about what it was trying to do for him. "He says it's pretty simple, his new girlfriend likes to go out with the running group for a beer after some of their races. Everyone orders pub food and drinks, and those are things he avoids in his own life."

Jim focused instead on his frustration about his weight and why he couldn't lose more around his mid-section. He recommitted to his food program, with which he'd faltered in the face of his expanded social life. Melanie related, "He says he knows he just has to be more disciplined about it because it's helped him so much with the anxiety and guilt he had about food and his body."

I asked Melanie what she noticed as she described her work with Jim. She identified a part who resonated with Jim's wish to lose more weight in his mid-section. "I really get why he wants to do that. And the program has been so helpful for him. His eating is balanced and healthy for the first time in a long time. Also, as he's lost weight, he's been able to heal some of the exiles who felt deep shame about being teased as a kid."

I observed to Melanie that she seemed to align with some cultural burdens related to food and bodies and asked her if she was open to exploring this. When she agreed I continued, "You said you've noticed a part in you who envies his fitness regimen and who chides you for not being more active. And now you're noticing one who is aligning with his wish to lose more weight around his mid-section."

Melanie challenged me, "I'm not sure it's unreasonable, I mean I think it makes sense to want to be more active and not let aging take its toll. It's an undeniable health risk."

I tracked parts within myself who could get seduced by this type of thinking and asked them to step back. "I believe it would be helpful for you to consider some of the beliefs parts of you carry about weight, health, and aging."

From the outset of my work with consultees, I emphasize the importance of getting to know beliefs they carry about food, weight, and bodies along many different dimensions: size, ability, health status, age, race, gender, sexuality, and socioeconomic status. Without this personal inventory, one that requires courage and dedication because we are so saturated with biases we've held for so long, we are destined to miss important opportunities for healing in ourselves and our clients. Melanie's beliefs about food, health, and weight blocked her from being curious about Jim's behavior and perspective. She assumed his fitness routine was healthy because she had parts who carried burdens about the importance of vigorous physical activity. Similarly, because she feared her own belly fat, she agreed with his parts' concerns about and focus on losing more weight. It was only when she acknowledged her parts and got them to step back that she was able to get more curious about Jim's experience. She realized, for example, that she hadn't asked almost anything about what it was like for him to train for the marathon or what different parts had to say about it and why. Also, until his new dating relationship made it difficult to sustain, she hadn't questioned him about his structured food regimen or wondered about what it was like for the parts who liked eating out with friends and liked eating refined carbs now and then.

The next time we met, Melanie reported having considered some of her beliefs about food, exercise, and health. She said, "It's interesting. As I reflected on it, I realized that I might have asked him more questions if he was a woman or if he had come to me for eating issues. It just seemed like these were positive changes he made to cope with his divorce and take better care of himself. I wasn't listening for the parts that he had to override to sustain this lifestyle, which is pretty rigid the more I think about it. But now I've been more curious, and that, along with his recent struggles, have opened up a whole new exploration of parts that need our attention."

Melanie learned more about Jim's fears about not running at the same intensity, his concerns about being seen as less attractive if he became less fit or regained some weight. Parts of him feared being seen as a failure if he didn't continue to abstain from flour and sugar or if he ate between meals. As Melanie explored these fears, Jim started to reconsider his rigid food plan and the parts who were deeply unhappy about having to forego flexibility and enjoyment. "I'm realizing the weight loss hasn't really stopped me from feeling bad about myself and my body" he said, "and being so careful is making it difficult to be with people as easily."

Debra and Amy: When "Breakthroughs" Go Nowhere

Successful eating disorders treatment often requires a combination of psychological, medical, nutritional, and psychiatric interventions. As I discuss at length elsewhere (Catanzaro, 2017), coordinating these different treatment components is often challenging. Providers come from different academic and clinical backgrounds and vary in terms of how they view eating disorders and in their comfort with treating food and body related issues. Communication between members of the treatment team is essential, as important shifts that occur in the therapy office often don't manifest in observable changes in food intake, mood, and physical well-being. The IFS model makes it much easier to understand and even anticipate behaviors that, to the uninformed, can appear resistant, conflictual, or extreme.

My work with Debra, a licensed social worker, and Amy, a dietitian, illustrates how helpful it can be when team members view the client's difficulties through an IFS lens. Debra and Amy contacted me for help with their client Jennifer, a woman with a long history of restriction and over-exercise in her early 30s. They had met during their Level 1 IFS training and were fortunate to live and work in the same town. Both women were aware of parts who felt frustrated and worried for Jennifer because of how much pain she was in and how she wasn't improving. Their shared perspective helped them stay aligned and aware of the current dynamics within Jennifer's system. For example, when Jennifer reported to Debra that the dietitian (Amy) was upset with her for going to the gym every day that week, Debra surmised this came from some polarization within Jennifer and not from Amy. Because she knew that Amy would not have judged her client's exercise-focused manager, Debra got curious about the outrage parts of Jennifer expressed.

Despite their close collaboration, Debra and Amy felt at an impasse in their work with Jennifer. They noticed moments when parts of each of them felt frustrated with the other. Debra said, "Amy recently left me a message about a session she had with Jennifer that felt really impactful, but then she proceeded to describe Jen's realization of how a critical manager had gotten her to override her hunger cues. At that moment a part of me felt frustrated with Amy because I felt like she was being overly optimistic when nothing much was really happening. We've heard this from Jennifer many times."

Amy said, "I felt judged by Deb and that made parts of me feel a little hurt and frustrated. We don't often have moments like this, so we thought it was worth getting some consultation."

Debra said, "I appreciate how Amy accepted my apology for being so judgmental. Jen's lack of progress doesn't make sense to either of us because she's been able to befriend her protectors and get them to step back so she can be with some of her young exiles."

Amy echoed what Debra noted, saying, "In one of my recent sessions with her she was able to negotiate with her protectors in a really loving way. She asked them what would happen if they stopped getting her to restrict and overexercise, and they said they really wanted Jennifer to be appreciated for who she is, not for being thin and athletic. We were able to go to a 7-year-old exile who was stuck at her grandmother's while her parents were at work. The exile was able to share how cruel her grandmother was. Sometimes she wouldn't let Jennifer eat all day. The worst part of it, though, was that the grandmother was all smiles when her parents came home. That made her feel crazy." Amy continued, "She was able to retrieve her exile, bring her to the present, and release the belief that she was unlovable because she wanted so much. She invited joy, hope, and ease to take the place of what she'd let go of."

Unburdenings like this made it difficult for Debra and Amy to understand why Jennifer seemed so stuck. "With her it's like one step forward, one step back. She cuts out a day at the gym and then walks 40 blocks to and from work. But in our sessions, she always seems to get somewhere, she has compassion for her protectors and helps them unblend, she reassures them that they don't need to do this for her anymore."

I took a moment and checked to see what I noticed coming up in my system. I was familiar with the challenging tag-teaming that eating disorder protectors often engage in – the looping back and forth that keeps the exile and its pain out of awareness. But Debra and Amy were reporting that in addition to this frustrating cycle there were also plenty of times when Jennifer was able to get to her exiles.

I got curious and said, "Something's obviously going on. If you can ask your parts who are worried and frustrated to step back, we'll be more likely to identify the obstacle." I asked them to describe their sessions in greater detail. As Debra related more about the session she'd had with Jennifer the week before, I paused her. "Do you notice how she often reassures her protectors that they don't need to do what they've been doing, that she can handle things now?" They both nodded. "The part who's doing the reassuring seems to me to be a Self-like part. This would explain why her system isn't changing. The unburdening isn't fully happening because it's being done by a Self-like manager who's reassuring or encouraging the protectors and the exile that it's okay to make a change."

Debra and Amy expressed relief at this realization. It can be difficult to detect Self-like parts because they mimic Self. However, they tip their hand when their actions reveal an underlying agenda. In Jennifer's case, it seemed her Self-like manager was intent on getting through the sessions without having to feel much emotion. Self-like parts are especially common in clients with eating disorders, who are often people pleasers who are afraid of affect and typically have years of experience in therapy where narrating parts are praised or pass undetected.

In a subsequent consultation Debra and Amy reported that their work with Jennifer had been very different since they started to track and help her get to know this Self-like protector. Amy said, "I realize now how I was mistaking this part for her Self. It's like a cheerleader or a coach. It seems supportive, but it's actually trying to push aside the parts who fear change. It's much easier to notice that part now, how it keeps us and her Self from really getting to know her exiles."

Debra added, "Well, easier in the sense that we know what's going on now. We see how that part has been derailing things. But another part can shame her for having a Self-like part. I've been careful not to let that distract me. Instead, I ask the critic to step back so Jen can be curious about the Self-like part and what it fears would happen if it didn't keep jumping in like that. While her eating disorder behaviors haven't yet changed all that much, it feels so much better to be present to what's really happening – that she has a part who is afraid to trust her Self. We know there are reasons why this part won't unblend more and that we just need to be persistent."

Conclusion

Eating disorders and disordered eating result from the complex interaction of protectors who focus on food and the body. Eating disorder symptoms are not bad, they're the actions of well-intentioned protectors who deserve to be respected, listened to, and loved. By offering a safe space in which to explore the different parts that get activated in their work with these challenging systems, IFS consultation helps clinicians become more Self-led and consequently more likely to stay curious and compassionate even in the face of perplexing or frightening symptoms. In this way the IFS consultant is like a torch bearer who passes along the clarity that within each consultee and client is a Self who knows how to heal, if only we can help them remove the constraints to that healing wisdom.

References

Be Nourished. (n.d.). *be nourished.* https://benourished.org.

Catanzaro, J. (2017). IFS and eating disorders: Healing the parts who hide in plain sight. In M. Sweezy & E. L. Ziskind (Eds.), *Innovations and elaborations in Internal Family Systems therapy* (pp. 49–69). Routledge.

Cox, J. A. R. (2020). *Fat girls in black bodies: Creating communities of our own.* North Atlantic Books.

Harrison, C. (2019). *Anti-diet: Reclaim your time, money, well-being, and happiness through intuitive eating.* Yellow Kite.

Piran, N. (2017). *Journeys of embodiment at the intersection of body and culture: The developmental theory of embodiment.* Academic Press.

Taylor, S. R. (2018). *The body is not an apology: The power of radical self-love.* Berrett-Koehler Publishers.

8 Making the Unconscious Conscious in IFS Consultation of Sexual Abuse, Sexual Offending, and Sexual Compulsivity Cases

Nancy Wonder

Introduction

Sex and Culture

In Western culture, sex as a commodity is something we are constantly exposed to on television, in magazines, via the internet, and on billboards. Having sex is also a natural human activity, yet it is still virtually a taboo subject and little talked about openly, whether between committed couples, casual sexual partners, family members, and even between therapists and their clients. Partially what makes it hard to talk about sex or sexuality is the paradoxical way in which it is viewed. On one hand, there is a message of sexual hedonism in that products are sold through sex, internet pornography makes sexual images highly available in people's living rooms, and being sexually attractive is revered and sought after. On the other hand, Puritan and Catholic roots in Western culture do not encourage sex before marriage and view sex as only appropriate for procreation. Being sexual appears to be one of the most polarized aspects of the human experience, and this creates unconscious vulnerability and shame for therapists and clients alike (Rosenberg, 2013).

Terms

Another aspect of the difficulty of talking about sex may arise due to the complexity and multiplicity of terms, and definitions of terms, in use. For the purposes of this chapter, please note that the terms *sex, sexual*, and *sexuality* may all refer to sexual feelings, thoughts, attractions, and behaviors. The term *gender* refers to socially constructed characteristics of women and men, while *sex* refers to those characteristics that are biologically determined.

I am a consultant writing about consultation. I use *therapist/s* and *consultee/s* interchangeably, with both referring to the clinician for whom I am providing consultation. Table 8.1 on IFS Consultation Processes, which are discussed later in the chapter, details processes that may also feature in supervision and will be highly relevant if you call or think of yourself as a supervisor or supervisee.

DOI: 10.4324/9781003044864-8

Inadequate Training Fails Our Therapists and Our Clients

Therapists and consultants, of course, have their own polarizations around gender and sexuality due to the messages they received from childhood, religion, and cultural mores. Without informed and adequate training, these polarized therapists' parts are likely to remain buried in the unconscious. Over the last three decades research shows that only about one-third of psychology graduate programs in the US and Canada offer sexuality training, and even this training is inadequate (Mollen et al, 2018). Without appropriate training therapists are unlikely to feel comfortable with approaching sexual topics with their clients, and this omission leaves the client feeling lacking in permission or too uncomfortable to bring up this sensitive and sometimes painful topic. The consequence is that sex is often ignored in client sessions due to the therapist (and consultants are therapists too) neither having adequate training nor having worked through their own sexual hurts, values, and beliefs about sexuality.

The inability and failure by therapists to welcome sexual parts and those affected by sexual abuse, sexual compulsivity, and sexual offending is harmful for clients. Research shows that one out of three women and one out of five men have been sexually hurt sometime in their lifetime (Koenig et al., 2004). Recent research also suggests that 56 percent of transsexual people experience sexual abuse or sexual assault (Grant et al., 2011). Moreover, internet pornography use is at an all-time high (Lehmiller, 2020), and couples struggle with dissatisfaction about their sexual lives (McCarthy & McCarthy, 2019). Therefore, the need to discuss all things sex related in therapy is paramount. Individual members of the Internal Family Systems (IFS) community have stepped up to rectify this paucity of information through writing on IFS and sexuality (Rosenberg writing about Rhonda in Krause et al., 2017; Rosenberg, 2013; Wonder, 2013). In addition, the IFS Institute has promoted teaching on sexual topics in the online continuity program (Schwartz & Wonder, 2019; Schwartz & Rich, 2020).

Courage and Vulnerability are Needed by Therapists Doing this Work

Therapists who do work with sexual issues must have courage and a willingness to dive down into their own vulnerabilities around sexuality. In addition, they need to obtain the appropriate training, face their own sexual hurts, and become conscious of their polarized values and beliefs around sexuality. The three case studies offered in this chapter illustrate how making unconscious parts conscious can lead to more effective therapy for clients. Each therapist has sexual hurts or beliefs that unconsciously impact therapy with their clients. One consultee was sexually assaulted as an adult, and another experienced humiliation and shame regarding her late development in puberty. The third consultee's father humiliated her as a teenager expressing her budding sexuality. Also, the consultant can have unconscious activation toward the consultee and client's work, as exemplified in the case in which my anger with end users of child pornography was activated.

Consultation

Before embracing the Internal Family Systems paradigm, I offered consultation in a classic format. My therapeutic paradigm at that time was based on my training in cognitive theory and psychodynamic concepts. Therapists would present the case, detailing age, gender, presenting problem, trauma history, and other factors that gave me an idea of their client's functioning. The therapist also offered their working diagnoses and treatment plan and perhaps talked about where they felt "stuck." Then we would discuss different techniques that might help the work move forward. I rarely went deeper to ask how the client was triggering the therapist or to consider how their work was triggering me.

Internal Family Systems offers a richer opportunity, identifying unconscious processes that are impacting therapy with a client around their sexual issues. IFS consultation helps the consultee identify their own parts that are impeding the work with their clients. These parts may have been hurt sexually, have many mixed messages around sexuality, and carry burdens or beliefs that, if left in the unconscious, could impact the efficacy of the therapy. In IFS consultation we are bringing the unconscious into consciousness by working with our own parts as consultants, actively working with the therapist's parts that are activated by working with the client's parts and working on parts activated in the consultation relationship. We then bring Self-energy, especially compassion, to these parts that might have interfered with the therapy process and/or the consultation process.

IFS consultation as I practice it (see Table 8.1) includes what I think of as an IFS take on the traditional presenting of the case. As a consultant, I like to ask my consultee for a thorough background of the client, including age, gender (and issues around gender), trauma history, presenting problem, and the consultee's perspective on the client's parts. The IFS consultee shares the parts of the client that have been identified thus far, such as managers and firefighters, and then the hint of vulnerability or exile energy that the therapist is noting. The treatment plan is always to understand the client's system, identify exiles, help the client form a relationship with the exiles, and unburden them as well as free the protectors from their extreme roles. Any diagnoses discussed are seen through an IFS lens as typical ways that protectors organize to protect the vulnerable parts of the system (Schwartz, 2017).

As the consultee talks about the case and where they feel stuck, the consultant tracks the consultee's activation around the client. I am listening for the consultee's parts that may be avoiding certain topics with clients, parts that are angry or frustrated with clients, and parts that might be intimidated or afraid of client's parts. Then, when a countertransference "part" is identified, I work to help the consultee to unblend from this part, such as

Table 8.1 IFS Consultation Processes

Case Presentation by consultee includes:
- background of the client, including age, gender (and issues around gender)
- trauma history
- presenting problem
- consultee's perspective on the client's parts
- any diagnoses seen through an IFS lens
- reviewing how the treatment plan is going (understanding the client's system, identifying, and unburdening of exiles and freeing up of protectors from their extreme roles)

Consultant seeks to remain Self-led by tracking own parts for:
- any that might be affecting consultee's relationship with their client
- parts reacting from own personal history
- countertransference reactions to the client and to the consultee
- parallel process reactions

Consultant tracks for consultee's parts, especially any who may be:
- avoiding certain topics with the client
- angry/frustrated with client or certain parts of client
- intimidated by or afraid of client's parts
- mirroring other parts in a parallel process reaction

Consultant and consultee work to unblend the therapist and get to know the activated part by:
- using the 6 Fs to establish Self-to-part relationship
- discovering if it is a protector or an exile who is triggered
- witnessing how the client is triggering the part of the therapist
- conveying compassion and appreciation toward the part
- encouraging the part not to do the work of therapy for the consultee
- encouraging working with exiles in consultee's individual therapy

Outside session consultant and consultee each reflect on consultation to discern:
- its impact on own system
- likely impact on the other's system
- possible impact on the therapeutic relationship
- what needs to be taken back into consultation
- what needs to be taken to therapy

---

noticing where it is in and around their body. Once the part has unblended, the part can begin to tell the consultee why this client is so triggering for this part. Many times, the part is a young protector that is doing the work of therapy for the consultee, at other times it is an exile who has gotten triggered by a particular client's part. Once the consultee's part unblends, the consultee is able to have more compassion toward it and how hard it is working to help the client. The consultee can then return to the client with more Self-energy. My understanding of the difference between IFS consultation and IFS therapy is that if an exile appears, the consultee is encouraged to fully heal the exile through their own individual therapy, rather than through consultation.

Throughout consultation, I, as the consultant, am feeling into my own parts for any that might be affecting the consultee in their relationship with their client. I might have parts reacting from my own personal history or my own countertransference toward the client, and these parts might be impacting how I relate to my consultee. My job is to remain Self-led and to identify any parts that are impacting the unconscious processes and seek therapy or consultation if necessary. Later in the chapter, I will show how being aware of my parts helped me provide Self-led consultation, which in turn enabled the consultee to provide more Self-energy to her client.

Working with Sexual Compulsivity and Finding IFS

I became fascinated by individuals with sexual offending histories when I participated in my post-doctorate residency in a state prison in Florida. I assessed all sexual offenders entering the correctional facility and offered a sexual offending therapy group. At first I was reluctant, then my favorite part of the job ended up being the group therapy, as the offenders who volunteered to participate were generally above average in intelligence and motivated to do the work of therapy. They were hungry for treatment as they carried a lot of remorse and shame about their crimes and were enthusiastic about completing therapy. I continued to work with sexual offenders as I completed my residency and started a private practice in my community. At that juncture I contracted to work with adult sexual offenders on probation and juvenile sexual offenders also on probation who were attending an outpatient program. In addition, I conducted psychosexual risk assessments for the Child Advocacy Center and the parents involved in foster care.

My treatment approach, at that time, was a traditional cognitive-behavioral model, which helped offenders take responsibility for their actions, identify thinking errors, and develop empathy toward the victims of their sexual offending. It was three years later that I met Richard Schwartz in an IFS introductory workshop, and my work with sexual issues and sexual offenders changed drastically. IFS helped me to see that when an individual sexually offends, it is because a part is acting out in order to soothe exiled parts that hold trauma. It was relieving to conceptualize this harmful behavior in a way that helped parts of me feel okay about and understand how I genuinely enjoyed working with these individuals charged with sexual offenses.

As I started on my inner personal journey in individual IFS therapy, I found my own exiles who had been impacted by sexual abuse by a beloved family member. I knew then why I was drawn to this work. Having been a supervisor of students, I became a consultant with IFS therapist colleagues. I also began to work through my past sexual hurts, reckon with my own sexuality in a world that objectifies women, and, in an on-going way, work with my own protective and exiled parts that become unconsciously activated around sexual topics.

I became more and more able to see the humanity of those that sexually act out, recognizing that they have been traumatized just as other clients have been. IFS appealed to me because it offers a non-shaming approach, treating the part that sexually acts out as a firefighter or perpetrator part (Schwartz, 2017). In addition, IFS emphasizes that building a relationship with inner critics that shame the client can help the polarized sexually acting out part to be less extreme. Finally, I found that treating the exiles that were impacted by trauma could eliminate the sexually acting out behavior altogether (Wonder, 2013). Over and over, I began to draw on this idea from Dick Schwartz:

> Offenders come to IFS therapy highly polarized and unable to exert self-control, and they leave with the inner leadership and compassion (for themselves and others) required to make amends and behave differently.
>
> (Schwartz, 2017, p. 115)

Case Vignettes

The following vignettes all involve some type of sexual compulsivity, not necessarily illegal. Each case shows how working with my own parts as a consultant and helping the IFS therapist consultees identify their own parts increased Self-energy, not only for the consultee but especially for the client. Each of these consultees had limited training around sexual compulsivity when faced with the issues in their practice. These cases are drawn from actual case material used with permission from the consultee involved. I have changed appropriate details to mask the identity of all consultees and clients.

I Am Not an Expert

Mary, an IFS therapist, presented the case of a 36-year-old, White, heterosexual male named Abe, who still lived in his parents' home and had never married. She said that she had seen him for 15 sessions, described the meetings as intense, and said that Abe described himself as having "heavy tension." She said that he had a complex trauma history, and his main complaint coming to therapy was not having motivation to accomplish goals in his life. Mary described Abe's protectors as harsh critics telling him he wastes his time and that he hasn't accomplished anything. Another protector was a firefighter who would look at pornography excessively. Also, Abe admitted that he liked to chat with 22-year-old women on the internet, and he gets aroused when the women call him Daddy. Abe's chronic complaint was "I am not living up to my potential. I am missing out, and I need a family and kids." Mary said that she felt stuck with Abe and often felt exhausted after the sessions. She described their work together as "going in circles."

Abe was raised by various au pairs since an early age because his parents were well-known medical researchers who would either work long hours or travel extensively. He was an only child and described his childhood as lonely. Abe's having told Mary that he visited dating sites to find younger women he could have casual sex with and that he looked at internet pornography led me to prompt Mary to further inquire about his sexual history. He admitted to Mary that he began using internet pornography when he was in middle school, and it was something he did daily, sometimes multiple times a day. Although he had dated, he had never had a long-term relationship.

As Mary and I talked about Abe, I began to notice that Mary didn't seem to be aware of the firefighter energy of the pornography use. I noticed a part of mine that sensed Mary might be missing the biggest variable holding Abe back, a possible pornography addiction. I observed that this part of me felt a little impatient with Mary because she was obviously neglecting this part of Abe. I asked my irritation to relax and then felt more curious about why Mary was avoiding this obvious "elephant in the room."

When I asked about why she hadn't been getting to know the porn-watcher part, she said, "Firefighters around sexuality are big and scary. I would need to be an expert on sexual addiction. I don't know enough." With her permission, I asked Mary to feel into the part that believed that, then asked the part how old it thought Mary was. "Early 20s," the part replied. This part reminded Mary that during that period she was drinking heavily and partying extensively. I began to use explicit direct access asking the part, "What else was going on during this time for Mary?" The part said she was dating a sex- and drug-addicted man, named Bill, whom she had allowed to move into her apartment. I asked the part directly, "What was that like for you?" The part replied, "I felt panicky and helpless." In an attempt to help the part notice Mary, I asked Mary, "Where do you feel this part in or around your body?" She said that she felt a warm, hot energy in her chest that was making her hold her breath. She then said, "This part is shit." I asked Mary if this was another part speaking, and she agreed, saying it was a part that felt embarrassed about that period of her life and that these feelings from the past were "shit." I asked that part to relax and, with the target part giving Mary some space, she reported feeling curiosity toward it. I asked, "Mary, does this part think you are still living with Bill?" At that point Mary nodded and began to open her heart to this young adult part. "She got blindsided by the severity of Bill's problems," Mary told me. Noticing Mary's Self-energy, the part went on to tell her that she felt afraid because there were so many secrets and to tell her what it was like when Bill had a psychotic break at her apartment. I asked Mary if she could make an intention to follow up with this part, and Mary said, "Yes, in my individual therapy." Meanwhile, I asked, "What does the part need until you can get back to her?" Mary inquired and replied, "The part needs to put away all of the bad feelings in the top drawer of the dresser where, during a fight, Bill put ketchup." The part put all the bad feelings in the drawer as Mary told me, "There are a great deal of bad feelings in there."

The part is an exile who holds trauma from that toxic and abusive past relationship. As Mary's consultant, I go no further than helping the part unblend and feel safe enough for my consultee to have some space from it when she sees Abe next. Mary will then follow up with this exile in her individual therapy. Mary has an ongoing therapeutic relationship with an IFS therapist where she can fully witness her exiles' experience, unburden the exile's shame, and continue with the healing process. The structure of the consultation hour does not allow time to fully heal exiles.

We then went over questions she could ask Abe about his pornography use such as:

- When did you first look at pornography? Research suggests that many people with a part addicted to pornography began viewing it when they were young (Skinner, 2005).
- What was your reaction to it?
- Were you alone or with other people?
- How did your use progress? (frequency, type, quantity of hours per use)
- What content do you look at? (male/female/homosexual/bestiality/sado-masochism)
- How does it impact your functioning now?

In addition, I encouraged Mary to include working with his critics and to take note of the polarity that Abe was experiencing between his harsh critics and his firefighter parts that kept looking at pornography (Sykes, 2017; Wonder, 2013). Eventually Mary will be able to help her client find the exiles that this manager–firefighter polarity are protecting. Like many individuals who get addicted to pornography, Abe was alone a good deal as a child and began to look at pornography to distract from his loneliness. The downside of this type of addiction is that it becomes a substitute for a relationship with a real woman due to the physiological and neurological changes brought about with habitual porn use, and masturbating to porn can even create an emotional attachment to the images (Maltz & Maltz, 2008). I encourage the reader to read the Maltz and Maltz's *The Porn Trap* to further study the hormonal and brain imbalances that excessive pornography use cause.

In summary, my knowledge of sexual addiction and compulsivity made me an expert that Mary could lean on as she worked with her parts getting in the way of working directly with Abe's sexually compulsive firefighters. In this way, I am lending my Self-energy to Mary so that she can explore her unconscious processes around working with this subject. My expertise and Self-energy provide a safe haven for people struggling with the challenging topic of sexual addiction.

Even Experts Get It Wrong

Lucy had been a long-time consultee of mine. One morning, she wanted to share with me how well she was doing with one of her clients, Fred. I had known Lucy for a number of years, being on staff in her IFS Level 1 training and then working as her consultant since that time. I knew her well and respected her as an excellent IFS therapist.

She began by telling me 68-year-old Fred's background. He was raised in a typical 1950s home, where children were seen and not heard. His mother had very poor boundaries (Lucy called her "boundaryless") and often asked Fred to watch her undress or come talk to her in the bathroom while she took a bath. She also shared her personal struggles with Fred and treated him much like a confidante, rather than as a child. Although the mother never touched Fred's genitalia, he and his mother would take turns "rubbing each other's backs," and the mother would unsnap her bra when Fred rubbed her back. This kind of behavior between parent and child is considered sexual abuse (Hunter, 1990).

Fred's father was alcoholic, worked long hours, and when home often became enraged and verbally abusive. Fred's perspective looking back on his childhood was that his father took his rage out on Fred because the father could see how close Fred and his mother were, and the father was jealous. In addition to the difficulties he experienced at home, Fred reported feeling as if he were an outsider, never really fitting in with the other children at school and in the neighborhood.

When Fred was about 10 years old, he found under his parents' bed some Playboy magazines that his father had left. Fred would sneak looks at those whenever he could and would feel aroused, not just by the pictures but by the possibility that he might get caught by his mother. The subtle abuse by his mother and his forbidden pleasure in pictures of nude women created a great deal of shame inside of Fred.

Fred continued to look at porn throughout his childhood and adolescence, and when internet porn came online, he found it fascinating. He had been married twice, and in both marriages his wives lost interest in having sex with him. He described them both as overbearing and distant. His first wife left him for another man. His second wife lost interest in Fred and asked for a separation. After Fred was incarcerated, she asked for a divorce.

In his mid-50s, Fred started going into online chat rooms to find women with trauma histories because he wanted to help them (which aroused him). He explained to Lucy that this is how he became imprisoned for downloading child pornography, as one of the women he chatted to asked him to find pornographic images of her that were taken when she was a child. Those were the images that Fred downloaded and then uploaded to send to her.

On the morning of our consultation appointment, Lucy was feeling good about her therapy with Fred, as they had found the exiles that were impacted by the mother's sexual abuse. I asked her for more details about his child pornography charges, and she admitted that she hadn't really been focusing on that, but more just working on whatever parts showed up when he came into treatment.

I could feel this tension growing in me. A part deep in my chest said, "I can't believe how this man is putting one over on her. She actually likes this guy! She needs him to take responsibility."

I said, "What about the child pornography?" Lucy responded that he only downloaded a few images in order to take care of the woman he was chatting with, and Lucy didn't think it was something he had done over an extensive time.

I literally could feel my part ready to explode out of my chest and said, "You need to delve more deeply into this Lucy! What part of you is avoiding this?"

Later Lucy would tell me that she could feel my upset. She said she had a part that was confused and surprised because my response was so unlike the usually supportive responses she received from me. Her goal had been to show me how well she was doing with a client, only to feel this part of me coming at her with some judgment and irritation.

Lucy returned to her client, sensing some ambivalence about how she was feeling toward him. While she sat with Fred, she began to be worried that part of her liked him and that part of her felt special because she was working with a client that many therapists would reject or avoid due to his criminal offense. She began to doubt her judgment and thought she was probably being naïve. Lucy began to question the progress she and her client were making.

Meanwhile, I was feeling into my part that had gotten activated in the consultation session with Lucy. I had an activated part who judges end users of child pornography. Even though I have treated many men charged with child pornography and even testified in court to help them get reduced sentences, this case made me feel the polarity within me that heretofore had not been acknowledged. One side of my inner polarity had gone to bat for end users of child pornography by offering them pre-trial treatment so that the judge would be more lenient at their sentencing. But the other, unconscious side of the polarity is a part holding anger toward both the creators of child pornography and the end users. This part has empathy for the children who undergo the humiliation and degradation of child pornography while simultaneously holding an intense judgment toward the grown adults that abuse and support that abuse of these children. Upon reflection and exploration of this part, I realized I was putting all of this anger that I had repressed during my work with users of child pornography onto Lucy's client. My part got activated toward my consultee's client because it felt protective toward Lucy. Moreover, this part that was angry was protecting a younger part of me that had also felt humiliated as a child.

In our next session, after greeting each other, I told Lucy I was sorry I was blended with a part in our last session. She looked at me with relief on her face and said, "I thought you were triggered by my work with Fred." I admitted I did have a part that was angry with Fred and wanted her to not be fooled by him. I then shared that this anger was my own part and that I was able to work with it. I then asked Lucy, "How did this impact you?" Lucy said it activated a part of her that gets triggered if someone sees her as "naïve." This led to us getting to know a part of Lucy that was a "late bloomer" in regard to pubescent development and had received ridicule from her peers throughout middle school. They would call her a baby or little girl, and she began to hate the feeling of being behind other people developmentally. I asked Lucy if it was okay to find this part that felt humiliated for being small, and she was willing and able to notice it, experiencing a hot flush on her face. I asked Lucy to spend some time with the part and asked, "How do you feel toward the part?" Lucy said she felt compassion and soon the part began to relax into Lucy's acceptance and love. I asked Lucy to check back with this part and follow up with her in individual therapy. Lucy agreed.

Lucy and I then worked with the polarity she felt in response to Fred, a part of her liking him and another part who questioned whether she should like him. I assured her that I would work with my part that is angry toward child pornography users and not interfere with her feelings toward Fred. We discussed her role as an IFS therapist with someone with criminal charges. I agreed with Lucy that it wasn't her job to "manage" Fred's behavior. He was in a Sexual Addicts Anonymous 12-step-group and was getting yearly polygraph examinations as part of his probation. Lucy admitted to having a part that was compartmentalizing Fred's child pornography charges because she knew it would interfere with her work with him.

Lucy continued to work with Fred, and, over time, he was able to unburden the young parts who believed that to be loved, they had to take care of Fred's mother how she wanted. Working with these young, exiled boys reduced Fred's firefighter part's urges to go online with women who it perceived needed him.

If I had not done my work in unblending from my angry part and apologizing to my consultee, this part might have prevented the healing of Fred's exiles. It might have unduly influenced Lucy's parts, who could have turned toward managing his firefighter rather than understanding the role of the firefighter in soothing Fred's hurt exiles.

Validating and Resonating with a Consultee's Vulnerability and Shame while Working with a Couple

Emily, an IFS therapist who I had consulted with in the past, called me for a session saying, "I have a million trailheads from working with this couple!

Please help me!" We made an appointment, and as soon as I saw Emily, I noticed the upset in her face. We contracted to begin working together while she saw this challenging couple.

In our first consultation session, Emily began to describe the couple: heterosexual, cisgender male and female, married for about 25 years. The man, Ed, was a successful businessman who runs a consulting firm, and the woman, Valery, was a stay-at-home mother who gave up her career shortly after she married Ed and got pregnant. Their two children were young adults, having left home to begin their own lives. Due to the urging of his individual therapist, who helped Ed see that he had a problem with sexual compulsivity, about a year ago Ed had come clean to Valery about his sexual addiction. Meanwhile, Valery had been in her own individual therapy due to memories of childhood trauma resurfacing. They had also seen a non-IFS couple therapist, who had asked Ed to complete a polygraph, after which Valery and Ed completed a "therapeutic disclosure" session where, for the first time, Ed was open and honest about the double life he had been living throughout the marriage (Love et al., 2016).

Valery and Ed decided to come to Emily for couple therapy because Valery felt that their previous therapist had aligned unfairly with Ed when he had described some of Ed's sexual acting out as "normal male behavior." In the initial contracting with the couple, it was obvious that they both had different goals for therapy. Ed wanted to keep the marriage and family together, and Valery was willing to work in couple therapy but was not sure she would stay in the marriage.

Emily paused at this juncture of presenting the case and said, "Why would she stay? I am curious why someone would have any hope that he will get better?" Emily shared that she had read the polygraph, and it was full of depictions of Ed's sexual compulsivity. She said that he had visited prostitutes on many occasions, had emotional affairs with co-workers, and masturbated to pornography sometimes three times a day.

I asked Emily if she could feel into the part of her that felt Ed was a hopeless case. Emily said she had a heaviness in her chest and solar plexus. As she tuned in, she began to realize it felt like fear. I asked her if it was OK to feel into this fear feeling in her chest, and Emily replied, "No it is too much!" I asked her to find the part that thinks it is too much, and she said it was in her head. I said, "Can you ask that part what its concern is about this strong fear?" Emily replied, "That it will make me freeze and clam up in therapy." I asked Emily if I could speak to that part directly, and with her permission I asked the part that was worried about the strength of the nervous part if it could feel Emily's presence and my presence. I also asked the part if it would trust Emily and me to not make the fear worse.

Emily said, "The concerned part has relaxed back, and now I can feel the fear again." I encouraged Emily to breathe into the feelings of adrenaline and tightness in her chest. She said that she was getting memories of her former husband. This part was remembering how painful it was when Emily found out, after six years of marriage, that he had an affair. Emily informed me that she had wanted to work on the marriage, but he left her for the other woman. I asked Emily, "Does it make sense this part is activated by this couple?" Emily replied, "Yes." She began to extend some understanding to this part and was able to make an intention to be with it another time. And for right now, this part and Emily agreed together that it did not need to help her in therapy with this couple.

Emily and I have been trained in the Intimacy From the Inside Out model developed by Toni Herbine-Blank, which applies Internal Family Systems work to couple therapy. One of the protocols used is tracking sequences, which finds out what protectors are in play when couples have conflict (Herbine-Blank et al., 2016). The protocol is initially a horizontal one, with the therapist tracking the protective sequence between the couple so they can recognize the protector parts engaging in conflict and begin to get a glimpse of the vulnerability underneath those protectors. The protocol then turns vertical, whereby each partner is encouraged to perform a U-turn back toward and down into their own experience, thus turning away from blaming their partners (Schwartz, 2008).

Emily expertly tracked sequences and found the parts that were polarized between Valery and Ed and the vulnerability underneath. Ed's protector wanted to have sex and be intimate with Valery, which activated a part in Valery who felt too much pressure and responsibility to be in the mood for sex. A part in Ed then got angry at Valery's lack of response. Both were able to understand the other's responses, and Emily helped them enquire about the protectors' hopes and fears. Emily asked Ed's angry part what it was afraid would happen if it did not get angry when Valery said no to sex. The angry part told Ed that if it didn't get angry at Valery, Ed would feel the shame of being unwanted. Ed could feel that his anger at Valery was protecting a young part that had felt unwanted in childhood. Then Emily turned to Valery's protector and asked it what it hoped for when it showed her the pressure and refused to take responsibility for pleasing Ed. It said it was vigilant to prevent hurt (as a child Valery felt responsible for taking care of her father so he would not hurt her sister).

I complemented Emily on her excellent work with the couple, and Emily's face began to scrunch up, looking as if she was disgusted. I asked her, "What are you noticing?" Emily replied, "I found myself feeling aroused when he talked about his arousal." When Emily said this, I was filled with compassion, having had that experience over the years working in the arena of sexual offending, sexual compulsivity, and sexual abuse. At the oddest times I had felt genital arousal when couples or individuals talked about sexuality. I suggested to Emily that this can be a normal phenomenon called sexual arousal nonconcordance (Nagoski, 2018). The idea that genital response always concords with the experience of wanting to have sex is just not true, especially for women. Genital response is an automatic response to something that is sexually relevant. In fact, for women there is only a 10 percent overlap between what a woman's genitals are doing and her subjective arousal (Nagoski, 2018).

I then asked Emily to check with her self-disgust part, and she said it had relaxed but it was still there. I asked her, "How do you notice this part that feels disgusted with your sexual arousal?" She said she noticed her mouth making a disgusted grimace and at the same time a feeling of being socked in the solar plexus. I asked Emily if she could breathe into this sensation, and she said she could and began slow, rhythmic breathing as she felt into this sensation of being sucker-punched. Emily said, "I am having a memory of my father yelling at me when I was 16. He called me a slut because I had on a short skirt with fishnet stockings." Emily proceeded to witness this part's confusion about her developing sexuality and her father's disdain and disapproval of it. I asked Emily to ask the part if she knew she did not have to do therapy with the couple? Emily assured me that the part now had a relationship with her, and it would not be in the therapy room with this couple. Emily also assured the 16-year-old part that she would work with her more in her individual therapy.

Conclusion

The purpose of IFS consultation is to bring unconscious parts of both the therapist and the consultant to the conscious mind through unblending. Establishing Self-to-part relationships with these newly-revealed parts increases compassion for each member in the supervisory dyad, which in turn leads to more Self-energy for the work of therapy, enabling clients to heal without unconscious agendas from their therapists getting in the way. I have the responsibility as a consultant to be aware of my parts that can get activated when working with consultees who are treating persons with sexual compulsivity. I need to be aware of my own exiles whose hurt might resonate with exiles in the client and/or consultee while also recognizing my protectors who can be angry with perpetrators of sexual abuse. This unblending of my parts can help me guide the consultee to more Self-energy and compassion for their clients. Facing our vulnerabilities and shame around our own sexuality will help us be more comfortable talking openly about sex and sexual hurts with our clients and consultees.

It is important in our work to have compassion toward those parts of individuals that can hurt others sexually or participate in pornography and prostitution. This compassion may ultimately lead to the healing of exiles who are driving the need for distraction from the pain of trauma from childhood. In summary, bringing the unconscious vulnerabilities to consciousness can lead to healing for consultants, therapists, and their clients.

References

Grant, J. M., Mottet, L. A., Tanis, J., Harrison, J., Herman, J. L., & Keisling, M. (2011). *Injustice at every turn: A report of the national transgender discrimination survey*. National Center for Transgender Equality and National Gay and Lesbian Task Force.

Herbine-Blank, T., Kerpelman, D. M., & Sweezy M. (2016). *Intimacy from the inside out: Courage and compassion in couple therapy.* Routledge.

Hunter, M. (1990). *Abused boys: The neglected victims of sexual abuse.* Fawcett Books.

Koenig, L. J., Doll, L. S., O'Leary, A., & Pequegnat, W. (2004). *From child sexual abuse to adult sexual risk: Trauma, revictimization, and intervention.* American Psychological Association.

Krause, P. K., Rosenberg, L. G., & Sweezy, M. (2017). Getting unstuck. In M. Sweezy & E. L. Ziskind (Eds.), *Innovations and elaborations in Internal Family Systems therapy* (pp. 10–28). Routledge.

Lehmiller, J. J. (2020, March 23). How the pandemic is changing pornography. *Psychology Today.* https://www.psychologytoday.com/us/blog/the-myths-sex/202003/how-the-pandemic-is-changing-pornography.

Love, H. A., Moore, R. A., & Stanish, N. A. (2016). Emotionally focused therapy for couples recovering from sexual addiction. *Sexual and Relationship Therapy, 31*(2), 176–189. doi:10.1080/14681994.2016.1142522.

Maltz, W., & Maltz, L. (2008). *The porn trap: The essential guide to overcoming problems caused by pornography.* HarperCollins.

McCarthy, B., & McCarthy, E. (2019). *Enhancing couple sexuality: Creating an intimate and erotic bond.* Routledge.

Mollen, D., Burnes, T., Lee, S., & Abbott, D. M. (2018). Sexuality training in counseling psychology. *Counseling Psychology Quarterly, 33*(3), 375–392. doi:10.1080/09515070.2018.1553146.

Nagoski, E. (2018). *Come as you are.* Scribe.

Rosenberg, L. G. (2013). Welcoming all erotic parts: Our reactions to the sexual and using polarities to enhance erotic excitement. In M.Sweezy & E. L. Ziskind (Eds.), *Internal Family Systems therapy: New dimensions* (pp. 166–185). Routledge.

Schwartz, R. C. (2008). *You are the one you've been waiting for: Bringing courageous love to intimate relationships.* Trailheads Publications.

Schwartz, R. C. (2017). Perpetrator parts. In M. Sweezy & E. L. Ziskind (Eds.), *Innovations and elaborations in Internal Family Systems therapy* (pp. 109–123). Routledge.

Schwartz, R. C., & Rich, P. (2020). *Self-led sexuality: An IFS based model for healing, pleasure, and empowerment* [online course]. IFS Institute.

Schwartz, R. C., & Wonder, N. (2019). *IFS treatment for sexual abuse: Victims and perpetrators* [online course]. IFS Institute.

Skinner, K. B. (2005). *Treating pornography addiction: The essential tools for recovery.* GrowthClimate.

Sykes, C. (2017). An IFS lens on addiction: Compassion for extreme parts. In M. Sweezy & E. L. Ziskind (Eds.), *Innovations and elaborations in Internal Family Systems therapy* (pp. 29–48). Routledge.

Wonder, N. (2013). Treating pornography addiction with IFS. In M. Sweezy & E. L. Ziskind (Eds.), *Internal Family Systems therapy: New dimensions* (pp. 159–165). Routledge.

9 Bias

How IFS Consultation Can Increase Awareness and Reduce Harm

Kate Lingren

Imagine the following scenario: A consultee with many years of experience, who you care about and for whom you hold respect professionally, presents a case with which she is struggling. The consultee reports that her client is struggling with his 16-year-old daughter, who he refers to as "defiant." He tells her, "She dresses like a boy, went to a barber shop and got a buzz cut and now wants to get a tattoo. I don't know how to get her to understand how unattractive this is. It was fine when she was younger, but now she has to see she needs to change if she is ever going to be asked out by boys." I ask the consultee what she noticed coming up for her while sitting with this client and even now, in this moment, as she is telling me about this. The consultee responds, "I really get his concerns." I notice some concern arising inside of me when I hear this. I ask her to say more and suggest that she "Take a moment and listen inside. What are your questions and/or concerns with this client?" She replies, "Well, I really want to help him. I understand his concerns, but I'm not sure what he can do that will really make a difference with his daughter. I did not experience anything like this with my own children. I was hoping you could help me around what he could say or do that would be most helpful to her."

Pause here and consider:

What are you noticing in your body as you read this?
What do you hear yourself saying to yourself about this consultee?
What is your first impulse in response?

Naturally, people come to us for consultation bringing their own parts with them. In IFS we hold the tenet "All parts are welcome," and it is an essential part of our work to ensure that this is, in fact, true. Helping clinicians to work with parts in their clients that hold biased beliefs is important, as is helping clinicians to work with their own parts that hold biased beliefs. In listening to this consultee, I am reminded that many times both present simultaneously; in this case the client and his therapist, the consultee, are blended with parts that hold similar biased beliefs, and I must decide how to respond. In fact, we must add another aspect to attend to as we hold all of

DOI: 10.4324/9781003044864-9

this, and that is our own parts that hold biased beliefs. Sounds like a lot? It is. I hope that this chapter will help both consultants and consultees feel more confident and able to welcome their own, each other's, and the client's parts that hold biased beliefs.

Introducing the Chapter

This chapter explores how bias, both explicit and implicit, and microaggressions arise in the work of supervision and consultation. For clarity, I use the terms *consultation, consultant,* and *consultee* throughout. The chapter also explores the responsibilities of the consultant to address biased beliefs when they show up in the consultee's clinical work and in the consultation relationship itself. I offer an IFS-based framework, BFOI (Bigotry From the Outside In), for understanding the role of biased beliefs in our internal systems and for accessing, witnessing, and unburdening these parts toward healing and greater Self-leadership. Fictionalized case examples illustrate the work.

Before moving on to outlining the BFOI model and the consultation process, I set out three essential aspects to this work: (1) knowing and accepting one's own identity, (2) understanding or engaging with the key terms and processes, and (3) the importance of holding presence in the face of shame.

Knowing and Accepting One's Own Identity

In discussing biased beliefs, it is important to know and accept one's own identity as a way of knowing what perspectives are being brought to the conversation; in other words, knowing where we are coming from. For the purpose of locating myself in this discussion, I identify as a White, lesbian, cisgender woman in my early 60s. I come from a class background of poverty, though I now enjoy the privilege of financial security. I identify as a mother, wife, sister, auntie, friend, and teacher. I am a clinical social worker with over 40 years of experience. I am deeply interested in implicit bias and how it impacts our everyday choices and experiences, and I am committed to working with my own parts that carry biased beliefs. I consider this an ongoing process that will not end until I take my last breath.

I have been practicing IFS for the past 15 years and have served on the Diversity and Inclusion Committee of IFS-I (the IFS Institute) since its inception in 2016. I am also a lead trainer for IFIO (Intimacy From the Inside Out), the application of IFS to couple therapy.

Understanding Key Terms and the Processes they Describe

Bias

For the purposes of this chapter, I use the term *bias* to refer to a deviation from neutrality. When considered in this way, bias itself is neither good nor bad. In this context, bias can even be prosocial; for example, when friends get together to support the local sports team. I believe that to have biased beliefs is normal and that believing and acting on bias, consciously or unconsciously, can and does cause harm when our biased beliefs are based on unfair and negative assumptions and stereotypes of others.

Explicit Bias

An *explicit* bias is one that a person holds consciously. For example, I have a bias that values shopping locally versus at online superstores. In the example of friends gathering to watch sports, each person is consciously aware of their allegiance to or bias in favor of their local team. In this sense, explicit bias for one's local teams can be prosocial and offers a sense of community and belonging. Explicit bias can also be negative and harmful, for example when someone consciously or knowingly expresses a derogatory belief toward or about a particular group of people. As I hope to make clear, whether prosocial or antisocial, an explicit bias is likely being energized and informed by implicit or unconsciously held beliefs.

Implicit Bias

An *implicit* bias is one that a person holds unconsciously. It is neither consciously created nor chosen and will likely align with messages, beliefs, and unwritten rules absorbed in and from families, communities, schools, churches, larger culture, and media. Therapists and consultants are not exempt from this process.

In IFS terms, implicit bias can also be the result of biased beliefs being rendered unconscious by our protective systems. Our protectors may take a moral stance toward these unconsciously acquired beliefs such that they believe certain biased beliefs are bad and having these beliefs makes us bad. The result is that the protectors exile the biased belief in order for us to believe ourselves to be good people. As is usual when working with IFS, what if we could accept that our parts have learned these beliefs quite innocently and that to them they make sense? The question then becomes What we are going to do about the bias we hold? rather than whether or not we have any bias.

Microaggressions

Whether intentional or unintentional, microaggressions are the everyday verbal and non-verbal slights or insults that communicate hostile, derogatory, or negative messages to people based on their membership in marginalized groups. These messages convey a sense of disrespect and are demeaning, suggesting that the person on the receiving end does not fully belong or is in some way fundamentally different from the aggressor, who is likely part of the majority group.

The result of a microaggression is to relegate the person targeted to inferior status or treatment. (Wing Sue, n.d.)

Consider the following examples:

- An Asian American, born and raised in the United States, is complimented by his college professor for speaking "good English." The likely hidden message here: *You are not a true American.* The likely impact: *I am a perpetual foreigner in my own country.*
- A Black couple is seated at a table in a restaurant next to the kitchen despite there being other empty and more desirable tables located at the front. The likely hidden message: *You are second-class citizens and undeserving of first-class treatment.* The likely impact: *We are not welcome here.*
- A female physician wearing a stethoscope is mistaken for a nurse. The likely hidden messages: *Women occupy nurturing and non-leadership roles. Women are less capable than men.* The likely impact: *I am not valued based on my gender.*
- The manager of a successful therapy clinic fails to act upon a complaint of racism made against an employee. The likely hidden message: *My therapists treat all people equally regardless of their race; it's just a misunderstanding.* The likely impact: *My perception is not trusted or believed; this clinic is not a safe place for me.*

Harmful microaggressions are usually delivered by well-intentioned people who are unaware that they have engaged in harmful conduct toward someone from a socially devalued or marginalized group. On the surface, these occurrences may seem harmless or trivial, but the cumulative effect of these daily insults has a powerful impact upon the psychological well-being of people from marginalized groups, eroding self-esteem and an already shaky sense of safety in the world.

Holding Presence in the Face of Shame

Looking at our own biased beliefs and speaking to bias in other people requires courage and a commitment to the willingness to be uncomfortable. Part of the challenge in doing this work is that implicit bias results in unintentional discrimination and harm. The shame associated with the idea that we have caused harm to another can be so strong that it prevents us accessing the underlying belief. In IFS language, when we have parts that believe bias is bad or shameful, our protectors will naturally block access to any parts that hold biased beliefs. These protectors might explain, minimize, deny, and even attack in order to keep us from feeling the shame of being a bad person. Being able to recognize and hold presence in the face of shame, whether internally with our own parts or when working with another person is an essential component of this work.

Bigotry From the Outside In (BFOI)

My colleague and friend, Dr. Percy Ballard, and I came up with a roadmap for understanding the role biased beliefs play in our internal systems and for safely navigating this potentially shame-prone inner territory (Schwartz et al, 2017). This roadmap enables accessing, witnessing, and healing parts using standard IFS protocols, and we call it Bigotry From the Outside In (BFOI). We arrived at this name as we realized how these biased beliefs are absorbed from external sources, that we are not born with them, hence they are acquired from the outside in.

In Bigotry From the Outside In, we recognize that there are layers of protectors that need to be acknowledged in order to access implicit or unconscious bias. The first layer of protectors we call "outward-facing anti-bias parts." These parts focus on bias outside of ourselves and have an intention of wanting to make the world a better place. These parts bring us to activism, perhaps by attending Black Lives Matter meetings or making donations to worthwhile organizations. They also serve to help us feel good about ourselves, locating bias as "out there" as opposed to "in here."

The next layer of protectors we call "inward-facing anti-bias parts." These parts hold the belief that bias is bad, and they may shame us for having any such beliefs. In this way they serve to keep any parts that hold biased beliefs exiled out of our conscious awareness. When we access these parts, we can then help them see that bias is a normal part of human functioning. We ask them, "If I did have parts that had biased beliefs, wouldn't I want to see them, to get to know them? Wouldn't I want to work with them to let go of any burdens so they can move through the world in a less pain-driven and pain inducing way?"

As these protectors relax, we may then access the part(s) that actually hold the biased beliefs. These parts are most often protectors, though sometimes they are exiles. A part that holds a biased belief is often a young part who is just trying to understand how to be in the world, how to fit in, and how to feel accepted and safe.

We then ask these parts who they are protecting, and, most likely, they reveal exiles who have fears or experiences of being hurt or not belonging. After unburdening these exiles, the BFOI process is reversed. We move back outward, checking with the protector that held the biased belief, the inward-facing anti-bias part, and the outward-facing anti-bias part to see how they are doing in response to the deeper internal work.

Working with Bias in Consultation

While training in BFOI is not mandatory for all consultants, all consultants will be working with biased beliefs with or without the training. My hope is that we can all begin with the end goal in mind: greater self-awareness toward increased Self-leadership in our roles as clinical consultants and consultees. Biased beliefs show up around race, ethnicity, age, gender, gender identity, weight, religion, class, sexuality, disability, profession, education, immigration status, and more. The question is not *if* these beliefs will present themselves in consultation, but rather *when*, and when they do, how we respond to them, whether from reactive parts or from Self-leadership. For the most part, in consultation I refer to these biases as "parts that hold biased beliefs." This language, while at times cumbersome, allows for the natural multiplicity of the human experience rather than defining someone by one of their parts, i.e., "John/Maryska/Li/Letitia … is a biased person."

Accessing, welcoming, and helping parts that hold biased beliefs in ourselves and others requires a great deal of compassion both internally and relationally. In consulting with other clinicians, we must be doing the work of welcoming and healing our own biased beliefs before we can more fully hear and confidently respond to these parts in our consultees.

In my experience, IFS clinical consultation involves a combination of parts work, mentoring, and teaching. In parts work, I invite the consultee to go inside, notice any parts coming up around the case being discussed, and unblend as necessary. In this way we discover what parts might be interfering with the work of the therapist. When the consultee unblends from these parts with the intention to give them the attention they need, the consultee is able to return to the therapy from greater Self-leadership. Using IFS, the consultant may work with all categories of parts of the consultee (including outward-facing anti-bias parts, inward-facing anti-bias parts, and parts holding bias as well as the exiles they protect) and through all the steps of healing. However, the process of unblending is often enough to return to the work with more access to Self and the consultee may choose to do deeper work with their own IFS therapist.

The mentoring aspect of consultation is of great importance to me, and something I came to appreciate more by what was *not* on offer from my own clinical supervisors when I was a young clinician. For me, the supervisor/consultant as blank slate strictly adhering to rigid boundaries in that relationship evoked a vulnerability that felt deeply uncomfortable and at times evoked shame, though at the time I did not have an understanding that this was what was happening. Mentoring involves authentic sharing of successes and failures, discussion about how parts of the therapist (including the consultant) impact the work, and modeling the practice of unblending from these parts in order to be more available to clients, all of which makes for a safer, valuable, and validating consultatory relationship. We clinicians need this kind of safety to be able to explore the very things that get in the way of our ability to offer deeper healing in clinical work. We need a safe relationship within which to explore our own parts – perhaps most especially when it comes to working with parts that hold biased beliefs.

The teaching aspect of consultation involves talking about what bias is (so we have a shared understanding) and that bias is normal and to be accepted as something we can work with. Permission to talk about bias is necessary and will be discussed under contracting. I also teach that expecting clients from marginalized groups to teach us/take responsibility for parts detecting for us is not acceptable.

What do we do about all of this? First comes acceptance that we all have explicitly and implicitly held biased beliefs as the result of the natural functioning of our human nervous systems and cultural conditioning. Next comes the taking of responsibility to educate ourselves about bias, biased beliefs, and the impact these beliefs have on marginalized individuals. The best way to approach this is in a context where we are not responsible for someone's healing; in other words, we cannot ask our clients or consultees to educate us in this area. We cannot ask people who are themselves from marginalized groups to help us understand when or how we exhibit microaggressions. I have been asked by well-intentioned people to help them by telling them if they ever say anything homophobic or heterosexist, as they would "really like to know." This kind of request puts the onus on the marginalized person to educate about bias and, as such, presents an (additional) unfair burden. As clinicians, we need to take responsibility to pursue the appropriate and relevant knowledge and growth through our own reading, workshops and trainings, educational videos, and discussions with others. Ideally, consultation is a place in which therapists increase their self-awareness, enabling them to avoid potentially wounding and unfairly burdening their clients.

In addition, the self-aware therapist and consultant asks for permission of the other before speaking about bias. This allows us to take further responsibility for holding how these discussions can be wounding and conveys that we honor the need for consent. For example, rather than asking me to police your language for signs of homophobia and heterosexism, you could assure me that you are working on this and ask me if I would be willing to speak to it were I to hear what sounded like a biased belief operating unconsciously in you or being shared explicitly. In this way, I am empowered to make my own choices around these conversations, something that may change from day to day or even hour to hour. It also honors the emotional labor required of me in this effort.

Contracting

Working with parts that hold biased beliefs in consultation begins in the contracting phase for how we are going to work together. Right from the beginning I intentionally contract with the consultee to work with parts that hold biased beliefs, stating directly that we can both expect and welcome these parts and asking for permission upfront to bring attention to them as they emerge and as we notice them. I also invite feedback from the consultee should they notice me speaking from a part that has a biased belief. Contracting in this way sets the stage for the more collaborative relationship that IFS allows for in consultation just as it does in the therapist–client relationship. It introduces and normalizes the notion of implicit bias and models the importance of the therapist noticing and tracking their own parts. By getting the buy-in of the consultee, we have created a context for addressing these parts in our work together, holding solidly to the belief that if not acknowledged and addressed, these parts can and do interfere with the clinical work. The consultant may need to provide some education to develop a shared understanding of what is meant by bias and how it functions in our internal systems.

Let's look at how these concepts can be operationalized via case examples. Again, all cases are fictionalized although they are based on actual clinical experiences over many years of practice.

Peter: Implicit Homophobia

Peter is a 58-year-old White, heterosexual, cisgender man with a strong Italian ethnic heritage. He came to the profession after having worked for many years as a teacher in a program for incarcerated boys. Peter pursued IFS training shortly after graduating from a program in marriage and family therapy. I find Peter warm and likable and enjoy the playfulness he brings to his work, which specializes in addiction treatment with adolescents and their parents. We have been working together for about 18 months, and during our first session contracted for tracking parts that hold biased beliefs.

Today Peter comes in and enthusiastically asks, "Hey, before we get started, who do you recommend for someone who is gay?"

I ask who he is referring to, and he replies, "Oh, I got a call from a gay guy who is looking for a therapist. He got my name from a friend of his."

"And you have no availability?" I ask.

Peter replies, "Oh, I do, but I'm not gay."

Pausing here for a moment as I listen to Peter while also tracking my own internal system, I immediately notice some tension in my body. I take a moment and listen in. I hear a part say, with some disappointment and some disbelief, *Oh no, not Peter too.* This part is disappointed at recognizing what it suspects is a homophobic part in Peter. I acknowledge this one and ask it to unblend so I can stay present with Peter. Again, I focus inside, and a part suggests, *Just avoid this whole thing and give him some names.* I ask that one to unblend as well and let it know that I actually welcome this opportunity to help Peter with his parts. I remind my parts that this is the work of consultation, that nothing is wrong here, and that Peter and I have agreed to this work. I then feel into my courage enough to respond to him, asking, "What do you mean?"

He pauses, clearly not expecting this turn in the conversation, and says, "Well, wouldn't he be better off with a gay therapist?"

Inside I hear a voice saying *He works with parents though he himself is not a parent. He works with women though he himself is not a woman.* I decide to allow this part to act as my consultant and to inform my response to Peter and say, "I'm curious about that. I have a part that is pointing out to me that you work with women though you are not a woman. You also work with people around parenting though you don't have children yourself."

Peter looks surprised, as though he has been attacked. "Well, this is different. Look, I don't want to spend my time on this today. I was just hoping you could give me some referrals. Or maybe I could send him to you?"

This comment brings the biased belief right into our relationship, given that he knows that I identify as lesbian, and I can clearly see he is triggered. I take a breath, ask my parts to further unblend, and then say, "I hear that this is not where you intended to focus today, and I'm wondering if you would be willing to spend at least a little more time here. I'm curious if there might be a part of you who believes that only gay people should see gay clients. Is that right?"

And I am curious now. I can feel my care for Peter expanding in my body.

Peter says, "If you are asking if I am homophobic, no I am not. You know my brother is gay and I'm okay with that. I told you how I confronted my dad about his homophobia, and that wasn't easy. You know I go to Gay Pride with my brother. I don't get what the big deal is."

There is clearly some protector energy here as he says this, and I notice my own protectors automatically responding to his energy becoming energized themselves. I gently remind them that I can handle this and ask them to move back. I remind them that I trust there is a vulnerability right behind Peter's protector, who could likely use some help. I say to Peter, "Okay, let's slow down a bit here. What just happened?"

He replies, "Well it sounds like you think I'm homophobic or something."

Inside I hear from a part of me that wants to jump in and assure Peter that I don't think that about him in the hope that his protectors will relax so that I will be safe. I ask it to trust me and to unblend. "See if you can hang in there with me on this, Peter. I'm not saying anything about you. I'm listening for parts that may need some attention from us." Having reminded Peter that consultation in IFS is often working as much with the parts of the therapist as it is working with the content of any particular case, he agrees to stay with this inquiry. I invite him to listen inside, asking, "Just out of curiosity, what if I did have a part that thought you were homophobic? What would that mean for you?"

He pauses, breathes, and then says, "Well, then you wouldn't like me or have any respect for me."

I say, "Because … ?"

Peter replies, "Because that would be bad. It would mean I am a jerk."

I respond, "Ah, no wonder that protector came up just now. It doesn't want me to think less of you as a person or to lose respect for you as a clinician."

He sighs deeply.

Here is an opportunity for education, and I tell Peter that there is no way he could *not* have parts that hold biased beliefs. I remind him of our contract to track, welcome, and help these parts so that they are not unknowingly impacting his work with his clients.

He says that would be helpful and then asks if he offended me, "You know, you being gay yourself. I really meant no disrespect."

I respond, "What offends me is the refusal to acknowledge biased beliefs and the unwillingness to work with them. Your part that assumed a gay person would best be served by a gay therapist is clearly well intentioned and does not offend me at all; in fact, many clinicians have a part like that. Right now, I am appreciating your willingness to take a look at this here with me."

Unpacking the Session with Peter using the BFOI Roadmap

Initially, Peter has an outward-facing anti-bias part. This part told me directly, "I can't be homophobic; I confronted my dad around his homophobia. I go to Gay Pride." This part serves to protect Peter by focusing outwardly on the biased beliefs of his dad. The intention of this part is to make the world a better place, and it helps Peter to feel better about himself by pointing out how his dad is biased and he is not, that he is "good." This part holds the belief that it is Peter's job to change his dad lest he be complicit in the father's biased belief.

Next, we can recognize what we call Peter's inward-facing anti-bias part. This part shows up when he says, in essence, "I'm not homophobic. My brother is gay, and I'm okay with it. I'm not a bad person." This part's job is also to help Peter to feel good about himself, but it points to his own behavior, separate from reacting to bias in someone else. Unfortunately, this protector often ends up shaming bias, thereby rendering it hidden and unavailable to access. For Peter, this part, which believes having a homophobic belief would make him bad, keeps him from accessing any parts that might, in fact, still hold some homophobic/heteronormative bias.

We can ask this part, "What if it were a normal human experience to absorb and hold biased beliefs? If I have a part that holds a biased belief, wouldn't I want to access it so that I could help it to unburden and unload that belief?"

More specifically, we can ask Peter, "And what would it mean about you if you had absorbed some homophobic beliefs purely by being raised in a culture that devalues LGBTQI+ people?" This question will likely access the shame that needs some attention in order for us to be able to move deeper inside his system.

Working with the relevant protectors allows us to approach the part that actually holds the biased belief, itself a protector. These parts may have picked up the bias as a way of understanding the world and how to be in it. In Peter's case this part watched closely who was accepted and who wasn't, what kind of relationships were embraced, and which ones met with negative reactions. This part likely took in that boys should like girls and that boys who did not were not normal and to be rejected. Perhaps this part's intention was to help Peter feel more solid in his identity, in this case by defining him by who he is not.

I ask Peter, "Okay, now, listening inside, can you locate the part that does not believe you can work with gay people? See if it can show you where it got this belief."

He is quiet for a long moment, eyes closed. When he responds, he looks at me with tears in his eyes. "Yes," he says. I ask if he wants to share what he is noticing, reminding him that he doesn't have to. Peter goes on to share experiences in school where he clearly got messages around what was acceptable and safe for him in terms of sexual orientation. I listen with compassion.

After spending as much time as needed with the part holding the biased belief, we ask permission to go to Peter's exile, a part that just wanted to fit in, be accepted, understand right and wrong, comprehend good and bad, and feel safe in the world. The exile had automatically and unconsciously picked up messages from the environment without the ability to consider these messages with discernment.

Once the exile was witnessed, retrieved, and unburdened, we then went back through the BFOI process in reverse. For Peter, this meant checking first with the protector who held the biased belief that he could not work with gay people. Usually, I find that this part feels relieved that the exile has been unburdened. We then go to the inward-facing anti-bias part to hear its experience now that the belief and the exile it was protecting have been witnessed and tended to. And finally, we check in with the outward-facing anti-bias part in the same way.

This process gets repeated for each part that holds a biased belief and can be done in a safe consultation relationship, in one's own personal IFS therapy, or in a combination of the two.

Louise: Personal Pronouns

Louise is a 45-year-old, Latina, cisgender woman who identifies as bisexual. She completed IFS training about two years ago and tells me she loves the model. In consultation today, Louise presents a new client of hers, a 21-year-old college student who told Louise her personal pronouns are they/them/theirs. In presenting the case, Louise continues to refer to the client using the pronouns she/her/hers. After a few minutes, I ask Louise what she noticed inside when this client shared their personal pronouns.

"Oh that. Well, I don't get it. I've definitely heard about this, but I've never had a client like her before. I keep trying to say they and them, but it's just too hard for me to do that. It doesn't feel right to refer to a singular person in the plural."

I ask Louise what she hears herself saying to herself about this client's pronouns. She replies, "It doesn't make sense, and I can't promise I'll be 'politically correct' in this." Consciously using parts language, I acknowledge these parts of Louise and suggest she asks them to unblend so that we can find out how this makes sense. She seems surprised at the request, as if she is completely blended with these parts, but she does as I request. "What do you notice now?" I ask her.

"Well, I feel a little calmer, less judgmental. But I still don't know if I can call her 'they'."

"That's okay, we're working on it," I say to her.

She takes another moment and tells me, "That helps."

I then acknowledge to Louise that for some of us the shift in pronoun use can be difficult, and that I experienced some of that myself at first. Coming from a place of mentoring and modeling the work, I ask her if she would be open to hearing from me around some of the things I have learned about personal or preferred pronouns. From this more unblended place, she readily agrees. I tell Louise that correctly using someone's chosen personal pronouns is a way to show respect for them and create a sense of safety via an intention for inclusivity. Just as it can be offensive or even harassing to make up a nickname for someone and call them that nickname against their will, it can be offensive or harassing to refuse to use someone's preferred personal pronouns. Louise is interested and I continue, saying that I have learned that choosing to ignore the pronouns someone has stated they go by could imply that transgender, nonbinary, and gender nonconforming people do not or should not exist, which is an oppressive notion. I pause again.

Louise responds, "Well, when you put it that way, I certainly don't want to give this young person that message. I hadn't even considered that my parts could have an impact on her."

"Them," I say gently.

Louise laughs and says, "Yes, 'them.' I'll work on that!"

"Yes," I say. "I trust that you don't want to wound this person, even unintentionally. Let's continue to work with the parts of you that come up around pronouns and if you want, I can give you some resources to explore that will help in understanding more about all of this."

"Thanks," says Louise. "That would be helpful. And thank you for not judging me about this."

Stella: Racism

Stella is a 40-year-old clinical social worker who has been practicing for 15 years, the first ten of which were in a hospital setting and the last five in a community mental health center. She is Black, of African American heritage, and identifies as heterosexual and cisgender. Stella had been reading about IFS and was interested in learning more about it and maybe taking a training. She got my name from a friend who is IFS trained, and this was our sixth consultation session together.

On the day of our session, I arrived to my office and our appointment dressed in very casual attire, something I had not previously done, having over scheduled my morning with errands and not left enough time to stop at home to change. We exchanged greetings, checked in, and Stella began to present a case. Shortly into the session, she stopped talking about the case and asked me about my shoes, which were rather worn-out sneakers. I happily responded that I loved these shoes and have had them forever.

Stella paused and then said, "If I had ever arrived at a professional meeting in those shoes, I would have been criticized and told I was dressed inappropriately."

My first reaction was to feel surprised and stunned. I then noticed some shame, which was getting in the way of my being able to respond from Self-leadership. I took a deep breath and asked inside for some internal unblending, which thankfully my parts agreed to. My heart opened further, and I said to Stella, "Tell me more."

Stella then shared that while working in the hospital, she once arrived to supervision wearing sneakers. The supervision appointment was right after lunch, and Stella was just coming back from a walk. As she sat down, the supervisor, who was White, indicated Stella's footwear and asked, "Are you planning to wear those while seeing clients this afternoon?" Before she could respond, the supervisor went on to say, "You are going to have to learn how to present yourself in a professional manner. Clients and colleagues are not going to respect you otherwise." Stella recalled how this was the first time in two years of working in that hospital with that supervisor that she had arrived to supervision wearing sneakers. She paused in her sharing, and we both sat in silence for a moment.

I then said, "I am so sorry that happened to you. It sounds painful and also shaming."

Stella responded that it was indeed shaming and said, "I still feel shame when I think of how she talked to me that day." She shared how she felt deeply hurt and misunderstood in that moment, assaulted really.

I asked Stella if she wanted to stay with what was coming up for her in the moment. After a pause she said, "Yes, I do. But I am finding it uncomfortable talking with you about this given that you are White."

I noticed a part of me that wanted to assure Stella that it was okay to talk with me about this, even though I am White, and that I understood how painful this was for her. Despite its good intentions, I let that part know that not only would that comment not be helpful, it simply would not be true; as a White person, I cannot possibly understand the experience of racism for a person of color in America. To say it was okay to talk with me would be minimizing the very real concerns of her protectors based on more than 400 years of racialized trauma. I asked that part to move back and just allow me to stay present with Stella, with nothing to fix or make better. I then said,

"I can imagine it would be hard to talk with a White person about this incident of racism. Let's listen to what your parts need right now, from you, from me, from us."

After a few moments, Stella said that she would like to go back to the case she was presenting and talk with her own therapist, who is also a person of color, about the still raw feelings of hurt, misunderstanding, and danger that were coming up for her. I agreed and said that race was something that would continue to be acknowledged in this room, and I was glad she had brought up how the way I was dressed had triggered something in her. I asked if there was anything else she wanted to speak for around this, knowing we could come back to it at another time.

She said, "Thanks, but no. Not right now."

As I reflected on this experience, I looked out for any outward-facing anti-bias parts coming up and noticed a part that felt highly critical of the former supervisor. I then wondered if I had done enough to create safety for Stella or if my responses had been less than ideal. I asked inside, "What if I didn't handle this exactly right? What would that mean about me?" What I heard from my inward-facing anti-bias part was that if I hadn't handled this *right*, I would have perpetuated racism and injured Stella, which would make me morally bad and clinically inept. In response, I said to myself, "Ah, okay, there is more work to do here," and I made a firm internal commitment to attend to this in my next IFS therapy session.

I then thought about how I had never had the experience of a supervisor commenting in such a way on my attire and, even if they had, as a White person, I would probably not have had to consider the possibility of racism in the interaction. I would very likely not have had to think about the potential for harm to myself, my employment, or my reputation going forward. I could have attributed the comment to misattunement and then, power dynamics aside, considered whether I wanted to speak to it or not. It is a manifestation of White privilege to not have to consider my own race as a part of my experience.

By acknowledging my "Whiteness" and asking permission to either stay with this or not, I was validating that not only was the issue of race in the room, but also that I was available to talk about it. I did not ask Stella to explain why the supervisor's comment felt racist, which would have been more about me than about her. A therapist of color would not need to ask Stella to explain this; they would know in their bodies the experience of which she was speaking. For our brains, which are constantly scanning for safety, "other" implies threat or danger. I believe that people come to us for consultation not to feel "othered," but to be seen for who they are (in all their multiplicity) and to be supported in working toward their goals.

There is another aspect to this case worthy of our attention. After this session with Stella, I had to ask myself about my own behavior, to do my own *You-turn*, or *U-turn* as we say in IFS: "Did my behavior in cutting the time too close to change before going to my office to meet with Stella have anything to do with implicit racial bias? Would I have allowed the same thing to unfold if I were meeting with a White person?" Sometimes these internal inquiries are difficult and painful in that we can find in ourselves biased beliefs that we may not want to see. I suggest we think to ourselves, "If I were to have an implicitly held biased belief, I would want to know about it so that I could work with the part burdened by it." This kind of inner exploration is actually to our advantage as clinicians, consultants, and citizens of the world. It contributes to greater Self-to-Self connection.

We Are All Works in Progress

My own journey of accessing, welcoming, witnessing, unburdening, and healing my parts holding biased beliefs has been profoundly meaningful, and it is ongoing. I continue to take advantage of the many resources and programs to assist in my process, including reading, watching videos, attending workshops and trainings, working with others, and engaging in personal work with a therapist who can safely guide the work. One way I found to enhance my own personal work in this area was to make a commitment to read only works written by people of color for one year. That year led to another. I read novels and non-fiction works alike by Black and Indigenous People of Color in North America. I read works by African, South American, Muslim, and Asian writers, including those who identified as gay and transgender. I read works by people who identify as fat and learned so much more about the impact of weight bias. By centering and listening to marginalized voices in this way, I have received an education that has been both deeply meaningful and at times deeply painful. Immersing oneself in lives and cultures other than one's own is one way to open up access to previously unconsciously held beliefs.

Every day there is more to learn, more to understand. For example, over the course of time it took me to write this chapter, I have changed how I use language in yet more ways. My appreciation for the damage caused by unconscious bias has deepened even more. This chapter would be different if written next month – more so next year. I am different as a result of this work, and my intention is that I continue to grow and change both personally and professionally. My hope is that you feel inspired to join me in this very important work.

References

Schwartz, R. C., Lingren, K., & Ballard, P. (2017). *Internal Family Systems (IFS) & Diversity and Inclusion* [Online Course]. IFS Institute.
Wing Sue, D. (n.d.). Microaggression: More than just race [PDF file]. *Unitarian Universalist Association.* http://www.uua.org/files/pdf/m/microaggressions_by_derald_wing_sue_ph.d._.pdf.

10 Keeping the Faith with IFS

Religious and Spiritual Parts of an Internal System

Mary Steege

"I'm supposed to forgive," my client Joe says. "'Turn the other cheek,' but every time she turns the other cheek he hits her again. I can't stand it," he says bitterly.

Joe, an Internal Family Systems (IFS) therapist who identifies as Christian, has come for consultation.[1] You can see why.

"What did you do next?" I ask.

"I told her God is a God of love and that God loves her. I told her Jesus never meant that passage or any other passage to justify abuse."

"I see, you tried to explain the scriptures to her. How did that go?"

Joe laughs wryly. "Not well," he admits. "She got mad. She said that divorce is not allowed, and women are supposed to submit. Her pastor said so. If she keeps praying for him, one day he will repent. 'It's worth it,' she says, 'if it will save his soul. After all, we're supposed to lay down our lives for our friends, how much more for our husbands?!'"

"Then what happened?"

"Nothing. Nothing happened," he says. "At first, I was shocked. Then horrified and mad. Mostly, I got scared. I didn't want her to get mad at me, and I sure didn't want her to find out that I'm divorced!"

This consultation excerpt highlights a common conundrum and some pitfalls that IFS therapists encounter when it comes to spirituality and religion. Joe got so activated by the things that his client said that he forgot foundational principles of the model and the IFS framework, which help us navigate such tricky waters. Joe stepped into the quagmire of content. It's compelling content, to be sure, with high stakes and real-life consequences, but when Joe got hooked, his own protectors stepped in and polarized with the protectors of his client. Polarizations that likely exist within each one of them are now externalized and enacted between them: parts to parts. Exiles tremble and quake; but no burdens are released. Not today.

No souls were saved in the making of that session, but we did find valuable trailheads, invitations for both the client and Joe. As consultants,

DOI: 10.4324/9781003044864-10

we can help consultees understand such challenging exchanges as opportunities – encounters that bring religious protectors into the light, revealing valid concerns that need to be addressed. In addition to any fears, these encounters reveal the hopes and dreams of a client's system: the desire of parts and the longings of a soul. They serve as signposts pointing toward the exiles and burdens that need attention – those of the client, yes, but also those of the therapist and even the consultant.

Who hasn't experienced some form of religious trauma or spiritual wounding? Who hasn't felt the sting of judgment, condemnation, or rejection? Don't we seek Self-to-Self connections at all levels of being – within ourselves, within human community, and within the cosmos?

Whatever our history, whatever our soft spots or hot spots, whatever hopes and fears we have with regard to the Holy, rest assured: IFS will help us find them and find the parts involved.

Religious/spiritual protectors can be daunting, but they have positive intent. Befriending them will make the unconscious conscious, the implicit explicit, and it will help us drop deeper into the heart – and the soul – of the healing process. These protectors are not obstructionist; they have legitimate concerns and can become valuable allies in addressing the existential beliefs, hopes, and burdens embedded in any therapeutic work. Once they perceive a shared purpose and once they trust in Self, these protectors often support the process. More than supporting, they may hold gems of insight and wisdom that help to guide us on the way.

As consultants, we need to help consultees develop spiritual fluency and competency as it relates to these protectors and the practice of IFS, and with this fluency, profound shifts begin to happen.

In consultation, Maria has been working with her overly responsible IFS manager that likes to run her sessions and manage the client's process.

"We're right in the middle of the classic witnessing/unburdening process," Maria says, "and it's going pretty well. My client is in a dark pit with her exile, but the exile is still hiding because she's ashamed to be seen. So, we're just hanging out with her and loving her up. We're sending Self-energy but nothing much is happening. That part of me is starting to get a little nervous and wants to jump in, but I hold her hand and that helps. Suddenly my client says, "There's a light!""

"A what?" I ask.

"I'm cautious," Maria says, "because my client has a strong manager part, just like mine."

"A light," my client says, "It's golden and it's glowing and it's coming closer."

"Next thing you know, the light is all around the little exile, and then my client is in the light with the exile, and they are all there together and she says: 'It's really amazing!' The exile shame gets absorbed into the light in some kind of spontaneous unburdening. Then all these other parts I didn't even know were there come and join in a circle. They're all in the light together. It felt like my whole office was vibrating."

"What was the light," I ask? (Sometimes even consultant parts like to know.)

"I don't know," Maria says. "I didn't even ask. I didn't need to. It was holy ground."

Indeed, it was. For a moment, Maria, her responsible manager, and I all simply sit in silence, savoring an experience of Mystery and feeling the keen privilege of doing this work.

Spiritual Dimensions of IFS

Internal Family Systems is a psychospiritual model, and people with religious or spiritual inclinations are drawn to it. They already know or intuit that healing and transformation takes place in the context of a trusting relationship or experience of the Divine. They may come rooted in a particular religious tradition or oriented more toward personal spiritual experience, or they may simply be drawn by the sense of "Something More."

In his article entitled "The Larger Self," Richard Schwartz (n.d.) notes:

> Though they used different words, all the esoteric traditions within the major religions – Buddhism, Hinduism, Christianity, Judaism, Islam – emphasized their same core belief: we are sparks of the eternal flame, manifestations of the absolute ground of being. It turns out that the divine within – what the Christians call the soul or Christ Consciousness, the Buddhists call Buddha Nature, the Hindus Atman, the Taoists Tao, the Sufis the Beloved, the Quakers the inner Light – often doesn't take years of meditative practice to access because it exists in all of us, just below the surface of our extreme parts.

People are thrilled, not to mention relieved, to find a clinically sound, evidence-based approach that welcomes the spiritual dimension: not only welcomes it – places it at the heart of healing. People from different paths gather together under the IFS umbrella, even though they may have no other affiliation. Some believe in a transcendent deity or deities; others think more in terms of energy and life force; while still others see self-to-self interconnection, both human and transspecies, as sacred; or some combination of the above. IFS may variously serve as an adjunct to current faith perspectives, as a portal for new spiritual vistas, as a faith practice of its own, or as a means for healing from religious and spiritual abuse and wounding.

Here are a few questions for a consultant to consider:

- How do you understand IFS as it relates to spirituality and religion?
- If neither spiritual nor religious, are you open and accepting of those who are?

- Do you secretly hope consultees or clients will share your beliefs or non-beliefs?
- What aspects of religion/spirituality might be difficult for you and why?
- Do you understand Self, in some way, to be universally present and accessible?
- Can you befriend a part even if you find its beliefs abhorrent?

The universal availability of Self is an essential element of an IFS practice. The ability to befriend all parts, whatever their beliefs, is a key component. Depending on your responses to these questions, you may have trailheads of your own to follow, and that's a good thing. There will always be opportunities to grow through the model, and even consultants need consultants of their own!

While it may help to have a personal interest, you do not need to be an expert on religion or theology in order to provide IFS consultation or therapy. You do have to believe in the model and trust in the efficacy of Self-energy.

Chris calls me in a panic. "My new client is a Muslim woman with a hijab and everything. She's having marital problems. But I don't know anything about Islam!"

"Well, Chris," I say. "Does she have a Self?"

"Yes."

"Does she have parts?" I ask.

"Yes."

"Do you know the 6 Fs and the 8 Cs?"

"Well, yes."

"Then you're good to go. Whatever you need to know, your client will teach you – about Islam, about her marriage and her own internal system. But maybe we should consider what part of you got scared and why?"

Chris got scared because she was not familiar with her client's faith. Even when we are familiar with a particular tradition, it's inadvisable to think we already know the frame. Even though we may share a faith approach with a client, they are the only ones who know the unique interplay between a particular religious context and its impact on their system. Clients are the only experts on their experience, and, if we invite it, they will lead us where they need to go. Encourage your IFS consultees to practice cultural humility (Tervalon & Murray-Garcia, 1998) to get comfortable with "not knowing" and lean into that great C quality: curiosity.

Chris needed to be curious about her client and herself. For her, consultation included a review of IFS basics then moved on to consider the parts in her that had strong reactions.

"Whenever you are stuck with a client," says Richard Schwartz, "There is always a part in the way. You don't know, however, whose it is – yours or theirs" (R. C. Schwartz, personal communication, November 4, 2020).

An IFS consultation session may include any number of different areas, such as:

- Regrounding in IFS theory and practice;
- Consideration/assessment of client's external context and constraints;
- Differentiating and welcoming parts of the consultee, unblending as needed;
- Discerning part-to-part interactions between consultee and client; or
- Applying IFS to particular topics, including religion and spirituality.

Consultees in consultation often gain clarity and insight about their own spiritual gestalt: their own parts, along with any beliefs or burdens; history and current context, including family and faith community dynamics and personal spiritual experience; not to mention the generational legacies related to religion that are so often intertwined with parts.

Here are some questions to pose to a consultee that help elicit clarity:

- How do you feel toward your client's religious/spiritual protectors? Exiles?
- What resonates and what rubs?
- Do you identify? If so, have any of your parts joined with theirs?
- Do you react against your client? If so, are any of your parts polarized?
- Are you aware of any protectors stirred up in you?
- Are there any exiles that might be touched in you?
- Does your client evoke anything from your own history?

Consultants can employ a variety of unblending and befriending techniques, such as parts mapping, interviewing a part, movement, conscious embodiment, etc. In the parts map in Figure 10.1, drawn from our opening vignette, we can see the protector–protector polarization enacted between Joe and his client, which mimics a similar polarization within Joe. We see aspects of Joe's religious gestalt, including messages from his past and current spiritual context as well as an IFS manager/critic. We also find an exiled part carrying a burden of shame.

No wonder Joe got temporarily tangled up in his client's process.

Through consultation, practitioners become familiar with their own religious/spiritual tapestry and unblend in order to remain present with their clients – even though the material may stretch across a wide variety of religious experiences and a client's beliefs may diverge from the belief system of the clinician. Consultees can learn how to language IFS as a spiritual practice in different ways in order to resonate with different clients. Some, for example, describe IFS as a means for discerning spiritual presence and divine leading. Others present it as a helpful contemplative practice.

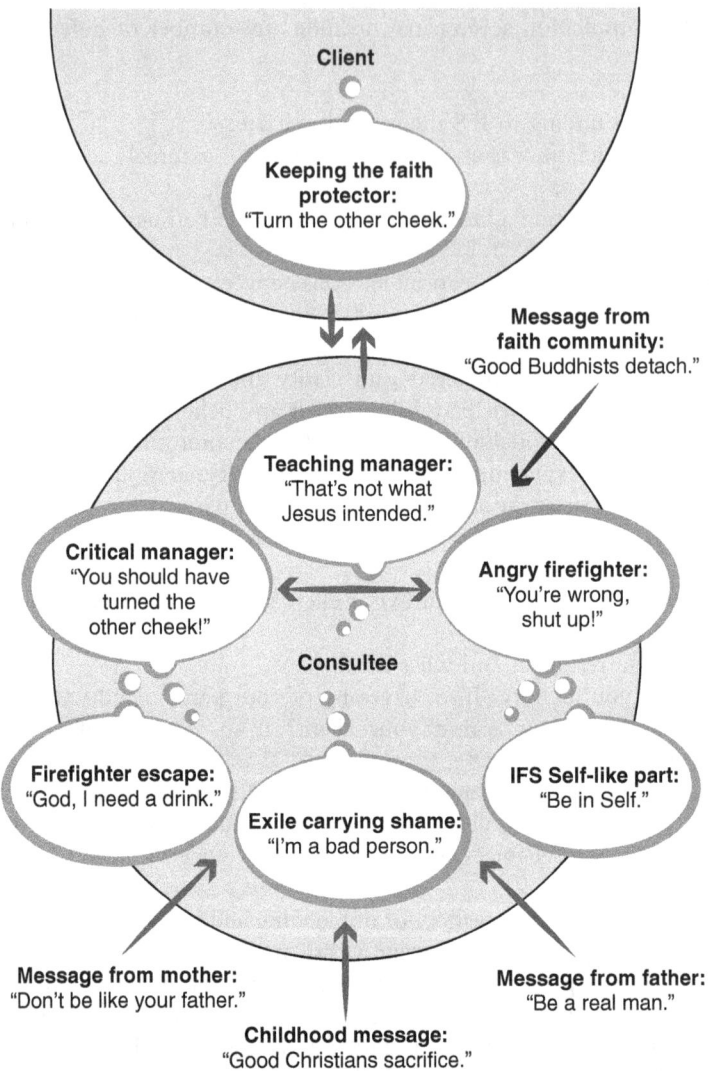

Figure 10.1 Parts Map of Consultee Joe

Many suggest IFS as a way to embody more fully the path the client already follows. Our consultees don't need to come up with a "one size fits all" formula in presenting the model. In fact, far better to encourage our consultees to help their clients articulate an understanding of Self that works for the client.

The practice in consultation of making links between IFS and one's own perspective will help clinicians, in turn, facilitate their clients in the building of bridges between an existing faith perspective and what they might find true within IFS. Clients may need reassurance that IFS is not a covert way to rob them of their faith but instead a practice that can support their spiritual development and transformation, which can take them where they already want to go.

There's another important area to consider with regard to spirituality and IFS consultation: when clinical work gets wobbly, it might be that your consultee has lost their faith in IFS.

Every spiritual approach has beliefs and practices; IFS is the same. IFS is based on certain principles that cannot be proven empirically – the concepts surrounding Self and parts, for example, and the notion of positive intent/ no bad parts. We also have specific practices and rituals which are codified in the 6 Fs.

When my consultees get stuck or feel lost in the work, I encourage them to go back to the IFS basics, bearing in mind the following questions:

- Given the framework of 6 Fs, where in the process do you think you might be?
- What category of part is presenting in your client?
- What part-to-part relationships are showing up? Polarizations? Alliances?
- What IFS exercise might be helpful in working with your client? Parts mapping? Sculpting? Externalization? Movement? Parts mandala?
- Which of the 8 Cs is missing or might be most helpful in your work with this client?

These are the nuts and bolts of IFS consultation, but at heart lies something that is, well, literally more at the heart: trust in the presence of Self. Trust in Self, both immanent and transcendent, both in us and beyond us – Self, a spiritual presence by whatever name we know.

"My client has no Self-energy at all!"

That's a common complaint. And this one:

"I need to be in Self with this client, and I'm so not!"

IFS is an experiential model, and we teach toward "felt sense" as the primary means for detecting the presence – or absence – of Self-energy. We let the 8 Cs be our guide. But when IFS clinicians don't sense the presence of Self, they sometimes begin to doubt and flounder. They blend with responsible IFS managers to redouble therapeutic efforts or with the frustrated firefighters who start to reject the client, the clinician, and even the model itself. They may join the burdened exiles in despair.

Consultants apply the standard IFS solution: unblend, unblend, unblend! But what if we can't? What about those times when parts are ruling the roost – in your consultee, in their clients, or even in the consultation session itself? When parts prevail, is all hope lost? It may feel like that, but these are times that invite us to trust, even when we can't perceive a C.

We have Self. Our clients have Self. Parts have Self. Parts of parts have Self – and so on, all the way down. The trajectory also trends in the other direction. Every constellation of human system has a Self – family, community, country, and so on, all the way up to world community and beyond. That is to say, we are each a whole unto ourselves, but also a part of other systems. The individual is part of a family, which is part of an extended family, which is part of a community, and so on. Structural family therapy refers to this as holons (Minuchin & Fishman, 1981). Others describe it as being nested in networks of relationship – picture Russian stacking dolls or fractals. Figure 10.2 shows an example of interconnected systems onto which parts, Self, and specific legacy burdens, etc., can be plotted by a consultee or client.

We are individual and connected, both a whole and a part of Something More; the transcendent, universal aspect of Self-energy that Richard Schwartz refers to as *Larger Self* – an energy that is alive and present and flowing in every client session, even though we may not perceive it. And, although Self doesn't have an agenda, Schwartz says, "Self does have a desire or intention ... which is to bring healing, harmony, balance, and connectedness to any system." (R. C. Schwartz, personal communication, June 28, 2020).

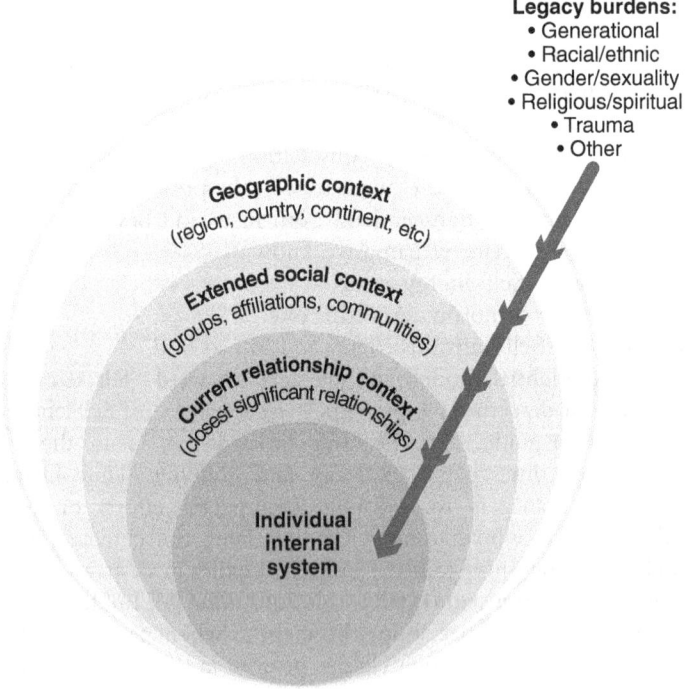

Figure 10.2 Interconnected Systems

Protectors from on High

Protectors can be fierce, and religious protectors are among the most ferocious of all. Devoted to the cause, they will sacrifice others and martyr themselves, if necessary. They may be feared and resented by people in the outside world and by other parts on the inside. The tough ones can be tough, but even the nice ones can be entrenched and difficult to unblend.

Why is this genus of protector so committed to their role?

Typical protectors organize heroically around issues of survival – real or historic or imagined; psychological, physical, or relational. Religious/spiritual protectors serve as "superhero" protectors focused on the ultimate survival issue – the saving or retrieving of one's soul, the achieving of enlightenment, the escaping of reincarnation. Whatever our ultimate spiritual objective, these protectors are here to help us achieve it, and they defend mightily against anything that threatens it.

Typical exiles carry burdens (beliefs, sensations, emotions, or energies) that arise out of adverse experiences, the big *T* or little *t* traumas. Becoming burdened happens to us all: the very people who are supposed to love us harm us, accidentally or deliberately. Consider then what it would be like to have these same experiences and subsequent burdens interpreted at the most elemental aspect of our being – within our relationship with the Divine or with reference to our place in the cosmic order. Exiles who experienced rejection from parents now feel rejected by God. Those who came to believe themselves to be unacceptable now believe they are unacceptable even in the eyes of Allah. It's bad enough to feel hopeless in a human context, but imagine feeling hopeless in an existential context. Such exiles pose a significant threat to the system. Religious/spiritual protectors will lock them away while simultaneously seeking their redemption.

No wonder these protectors are so fierce! They are charged with the keeping of our eternal spiritual well-being and that of others. The stakes couldn't be any higher. Given that level of responsibility, they do whatever it takes.

In her book, *Leaving the Witness*, Scorah (2020) explains her participation in the sacrificial culture of the Jehovah Witness:

> We were very invested in the trade-off we had made. We gave up any hope of a career, or education, financial security, and certain relationships, all for the sake of saving people, and goddammit – no pun intended – we were very concerned about their impending destruction … I derived meaning from the busy activity of my life and from my friends in the close community of fellow preachers around me. The organization and these people and this service were what held my life in place … I had been trained from birth to never stray from this hub of belief, this safety. My life depended on it.
>
> (pp. 4–5)

Regardless of how they may present, spiritual/religious protectors deserve our respect and compassion. Henry Wadsworth Longfellow (1857, p. 452) wrote: "If we could read the secret history of our enemies, we should find in each man's life sorrow and suffering enough to disarm all hostility." In the same way, witnessing the secret life of protectors can not only disarm, but bring about compassion and open space for healing and transformation. Religious protectors hold a wealth of information about messages given and received, of meaning made explicitly or implicitly. They hold important information about external context – the constraints and real-world risks to clients if they begin to heal and change from the inside out. They know the hopes and dreams.

We want consultees to achieve positive regard for all manner of religious/ spiritual protectors. Unfortunately, consultees may polarize with or align with the religious protectors of their clients without even realizing it. Personal beliefs and burdens create blind spots in clinicians. Confronted with a client's internal divide, it is tempting for therapists to take sides. We, as consultants, have similar blind spots and, without awareness, may enter the fray. However, it is important for the whole of a client's system to help everyone unblend and befriend – to welcome and treat protectors around religion with respect and honor. Already sensitive to judgment, rejection, and shame for where they've been or what they believe, clients don't need any more from us and will be on the lookout for it. Clients need a clinician who honors the whole of a spiritual journey, regardless of where that path has led or where that path might go. When practitioners facilitate a safe container, then clients are free to go where they need to go – to wrestle with their own demons, work through their own betrayals, and savor their own profound experiences of the sacred.

As consultants, we provide that same safe space for those seeking consultation. When consultees get activated around religious issues, we welcome all their parts, including the extreme. Even IFS practitioners can have parts with strong reactions related to religion or spirituality. No need to judge the judgers or shame the shamers or blame the blamers. If parts are really riled, we can even release the agenda to unblend. We simply welcome every part to the conversation, listening and befriending until these protectors get their needs met and their concerns addressed. Once satisfied, more Self-energy will emerge. The more consultees have the experience of having their parts and polarizations befriended, the more they can befriend their own parts on the inside, and the more they will be able to help their clients befriend similar parts and polarizations in themselves.

Who's Protecting Whom?

Protectors protect. That's what they do.

Religious/spiritual protectors operate in the realm of religion, spirituality, and morality. They may be driven by burdens and polarized with other

Table 10.1 Spiritual and Religious Protectors

Keeping the Faith Parts:	Freedom Fighter Parts:	Moral Behavior or Moralistic Parts:	Spirit-like Parts:
• Defend doctrines, beliefs, behaviors, and practices • Seek safety through boundaries and belonging • Have concerns about purity and contamination • Hold loyalty to the group over needs of the individual • May have tribal legacy burdens • May keep people in abusive, addictive, or unhealthy relationship	• Polarize with religious managers • Present within religious traditions as reformers or prophets; outside those traditions as atheist, "spiritual, but not religious," political activists • May be against any organized religion or community • Protect parts or people they see as vulnerable while overlooking own exiles • Escalate conflict	• Focus on behavior: personal morality or community ethics • May or may not be tied to a formal belief system • Do right and live justly • Breed perfectionism, scrupulosity, self-righteousness, judgment of self and others • Reinforce burdens of hopelessness, inadequacy, failure, shame	• Similar to Self-like parts • Spiritually syntonic with person's faith perspective • Maintain self-image of oneself as "good" or "faithful" • Focus on others but unconsciously motivated by personal discomfort • Manifest any of the 8 Cs or other religious attributes • Include parts that are nice, helping, rescuing, people-pleasing • May use spiritual practices to numb, distract or avoid

(Continued)

Table 10.1 (Cont.)

"The Nice One" Parts:	Spiritualizing/Spiritual Bypass Parts:	Predator Parts:	Parts Who See IFS as The New Plan for Salvation:
• Helpful and compliant, they use people-pleasing as a strategy for safety and connection	• Provide spiritual perspectives to help us "rise above it," seek ascending path	• Strategically co-opt theology or insinuate themselves into spiritual community	• Drive search for healing through IFS, become rigid
• Sacrifice own needs for others and can lean toward co-dependency	• Separate us from any challenging aspect of the human condition	• Garner trust and gain access to vulnerable people	• Hold strong agenda for change/healing/transformation through unburdening
• Managers or firefighters	• Well-intentioned but exile other parts and body in the process	• May present as part of manager–firefighter polarizations or within manager–firefighter alliances	• Polarized with other protectors that sense agenda and distrust drive for redemption
• Often undetected and overlooked by therapists because … well, nice	• Can evoke guilt, shame, experience of invisibility or invalidation	• Objectify and use others instrumentally	• May communicate "not good enough" to other parts, other people

parts, but they can also have authentic intuitions and valuable spiritual acuity. They know the longings of Self for Self and sense the system's yearning for internal healing and shalom. Though they may be going about it in the wrong way, these parts are doing what they can to help us reconnect with the animating life force that we may know variously as "Self" or "Love" or "God." These parts seek our good.

We can't fully know a part until we befriend it, but we can help our consultees become conversant with some common categories of religious/spiritual protectors (see Table 10.1).

Polarization and the Spiritual Divide

A nugget from high school physics: for every action there is an equal and opposite reaction. This applies to the physics of internal family relationships as well.

For every strong firefighter there is an equally entrenched manager; for every skilled manager, an evenly matched firefighter. Too many cooks in the church kitchen, too many protectors on a project and next thing you know, there's a struggle for power and control. Conflict is a fact of life, inside and out, but we live in a culture that values unity of purpose and singleness of mind, sees like-mindedness as the primary means for building and maintaining community.

Spiritual people are often taught to avoid conflict. That, or to conquer it. When it comes to religious beliefs and behaviors, we may be expected (and expect ourselves) to be 100 percent in our conviction and our commitment. To achieve this, we try to repress, deny, or otherwise exile any parts that we consider to be problematic. Since we can't eliminate parts, efforts to dominate and control them only lead to increasing inner turmoil, not to mention guilt and shame.

The principle of multiplicity has been a godsend (pun intended) for many, a gift for clients failing to realize their own ideals. There is another way. Instead of exiling our parts or beating them into submission, religious clients can befriend them and learn to work with them skillfully – come to appreciate them, even those they once reviled.

Some therapists, however, inadvertently align with the manager parts of clients and managerial agenda for change in the hope that clients will live right and feel better. Other therapists align with firefighter energy, fanning the flames of rebellion out of a personal agenda for liberation. We can get inducted into our client's internal system, especially polarizations about moral/spiritual/religious issues. A key feature of IFS consultation is to help consultees see where they got sucked in and why. We can ask consultees these questions:

- What parts of your client are at play around this issue?
- Do you have strong opinions about this issue?

- Do you agree with any of your client's parts?
- Do you react against any of them?
- Is your client experiencing a polarization and, if so, have you taken sides?

In addition to offering questions, you might ask your consultee to map their own parts related to this issue, the client's parts related to this issue, and the interplay of both, as we saw previously in the map of Joe's system (Figure 10.1).

The Exiling of Protectors

In many polarizations, protective parts are evenly matched. A manager may be in control for longer periods of time, but then firefighters rebel and temporarily overthrow the regime through intensity and acting out behaviors. Power and influence get redistributed and equalized through a kind of checks-and-balances cycle that repeats.

In other systems, it's not so much a polarization as a domination – one part, or an alliance of parts, consistently rules the roost. In some people, managers have a totalitarian grip, but in others, rebel forces bust out all over.

Institutions and organizations, ideologies and theologies, any plan for salvation or self-improvement – these are the natural playgrounds for managers with their gifts of logic and long-term thinking, their skills in strategy and structure. One common goal of the religious life has been to put "reason" in charge of "passions" – to privilege the mind over the body. No wonder people who identify as religious or spiritual often have an abundance of managers, though it is important to note that manager parts themselves can be spiritually problematic. Socially acceptable, highly esteemed, and rewarded in our culture, they typically have issues with trust and control. They don't trust the Self of a person, and they don't trust the leadership of a Higher Power.

Firefighters, on the other hand, are not, for the most part, socially acceptable. People whose systems are dominated by addictive, angry, or dissociative firefighters are often criticized and reviled for the destruction that lies in their wake. Judged as sinful and immoral, seen as lacking in self-discipline and self-control, or considered defective in character, firefighters do not come to the regularly scheduled religious gatherings, but they do attend the 12-step meetings housed in basement rooms below.

Multi-partiality (Sutherland, 2005) is a concept from family systems theory in which therapists recognize and affirm the value and role played by every family member – no room for favorites, no reason to judge among them. Similarly, from the internal family systems perspective, managers are not inherently better than firefighters. They are both protectors focused on getting the job done; they just do the job in different ways. Both are forms of protector energy that exile the exiles and obscure the leadership of Self.

In our eagerness to get to those parts we know as "exiles," we can easily overlook the ways in which protectors themselves get *exiled*, especially those labeled as "bad" from within the context of a particular religious or spiritual framework. Where intellect is privileged over emotion, intensely feeling firefighters are exiled. In others, where emotion is prized over the intellect, reasoning managers are suspect. In many paths, obedient parts are seen as superior to those who question and doubt. This approach creates a natural insider/outside orientation.

As consultants, we want our clinicians to understand the exiling process as it pertains to *protectors* and then teach them how to draw out this dynamic for their own clients to see and consider. Here are a couple of approaches to use both in consultation and in the therapy relationship that elicit this kind of conversation:

What does it mean to be a good/faithful Jew (Muslim, Buddhist, person, etc.)?

Complete these sentences:

(a)   A good Catholic is _____?
(b)   A good Catholic does not _____?

You'll be surprised how quickly clients answer. Parts know!

Follow-up questions to flesh this out:

- How do you know all this?
- How did you learn it? From whom?
- If this is what it means to be good, what does bad look like?
- And what happens to the "bad" ones?
- Are there good and bad parts of you?
- How do you feel toward the "bad" parts? What do you do with them?

Once we understand the context and concerns for exiling protectors, we can then address the fears that drive it, just as we would take seriously and compassionately address the fears of any protector.

Particularly poignant, the process of exiling "bad" protectors for the sake of remaining spiritually safe can end up reinforcing experiences of trauma and perpetuate victimization. It can crush the soul.

Diana Butler Bass (2018) describes how this dynamic played out in her own quest for healing following sexual abuse:

[M]y search for freedom from the pain led me to a fundamentalist church, a community of clear-cut rules and gender roles, with rigid boundaries, a place where I thought no one could hurt me again. Although I did not fully comprehend it at the time, its spiritual safety came with a price – the requirements of forgiveness and a cheerful piety of gratitude. ... This is where I felt stuck: The fear was real, and it was not my fault. How to get rid of something you neither created nor deserved? What if you are afraid because your room was not safe at night? What if you are angry because no one was protecting you from harm? What if you mourn the loss of your sense of personhood? These are not just "negative" emotions. They are genuine feelings induced by trauma. They are natural responses when pain is inflicted on you – how much worse would it be if a victim did not feel fear, anger, and grief? … gratitude can be difficult, especially if we sought refuge in religious communities that reinforced shame under the guise of salvation.

Butler Bass came to see the positive intent of her parts, even the ones with rage. In other people, these parts do not fare so well.

Colleen presents her twenty-something client, a single woman who identifies as Catholic and is racked with guilt over her sexual encounters with men. Colleen talks about her client's situation for a while, and then I facilitate a U-turn of her own.

"What's your issue in all this?" I ask, "What is leading you to bring this particular case for consultation?"

She considers. "I get confused," she says. "I personally don't think it's wrong if she wants to have sex even if she's not married, but it *is* causing a lot of problems with her mother. And it makes her feel bad about herself. She says she wants to be a good Catholic and stop doing it, and, to be honest, she's putting herself in some really unsafe situations. She might even have a sex addiction. So, what am I supposed to do? I know all parts are welcome but at the same time, I feel like she really needs to stop!"

Colleen has gotten hooked by her client's internal debate. Understandably. It's a sensitive dilemma and comes with consequences. Colleen can feel herself starting to fall in line with a manager-driven agenda – that of her client's managers, the client's mother's managers, and those of the church and community. It's a lot of pressure for a client, and a lot of pressure on a therapist.

We talk a little about the behavior-focused religious protectors and corresponding firefighter behavior. I remind Colleen that she has the capacity to welcome and support all of her client's parts and their perspectives. She doesn't have to decide which one is right. At this beginning stage of the process, Collen can help her client flesh out the polarization, then begin a process of shuttle diplomacy. She can start by exploring more fully the context of the manager that brought the client into counseling in the first place, asking her:

- What does it mean to be a good Catholic?
- Where does sex fit in?
- How do you know all this? Where did you learn it and from whom?
- What are the consequences of not being a good Catholic?

Then we role-play invitations that might help clients get curious toward the "acting out" firefighter. Colleen's version ends up something like this: "Part of you wants to stop sleeping around, but then there's this other part of you that doesn't want to stop, doesn't seem to care about being a good Catholic, and this whole thing is causing you a lot of problems. Is that right?

"What if we could get to know that 'having sex' part a little better and see what's going on there, learn what's underneath all that?

"I suspect the part that keeps you having sex has got some reason for doing what it's doing. It might be good to know what that's about."

Next session, Colleen reports that the "bad" part of her client did, in fact, have a positive intent. It wanted her to feel good, even if just for a little while. The strategy isn't playing out well over time, but once the client could see the positive intent of this "bad" part, she softened toward it. Now she's interested in the next step: exploring what it is that makes her feel so bad in the first place.

Not once does Colleen have to take sides in the moral debate. She doesn't have to manage a client's manager or fight with the client's firefighter. Befriending the protectors doesn't mean we condone what they do; it does mean we show care for them even though they are doing what they do. Colleen helped facilitate a trusting relationship between the client's Self and both protectors, which, in turn, made room for more Self-leadership in the system, allowing exiles to heal and inner consensus to emerge.

In systems that are skewed, where a protective energy has been exiled, whether firefighter or managerial, we want to welcome these protectors back into relationship with Self. Treasured for the gifts they bring and honored for their contributions to the whole, they willingly give up the roles that are no longer needed and no longer fit. They are glad to know that Self-leadership is in place and on the job.

Off the IFS Map

Sometimes consultees bring into consultation sessions spiritual dimensions that deviate from the traditional 6 Fs framework: clients who incorporate religious material into the work or past life unburdening, or an unexpected, unexplained spiritual phenomenon occurs.

Those who provide consultation need to be comfortable with these kinds of experiences and know how to support consultees when sessions go off the IFS map. We want to equip our consultees so they can welcome a manifold of religious practices or divine manifestations while, at the same time, discerning the presence of any protectors in the mix (their own and that of the client).

When clients want to incorporate elements from their faith approach, we honor this, so long as it feels like the leading of Self. We can coach IFS practitioners on various ways to differentiate between possible origins of that desire, having them ask the client:

- Is that suggestion coming from the target part or could it be another part with an idea about what needs to happen?
- What kind of reaction do you get inside when you suggest this element?
- How does the target part feel about including that element?
- Does the suggestion feel like it is coming from a part, or something else?

For example, the client says, "This little boy needs to be anointed!" Our consultee can inquire, "Is that coming from the little boy, from another part that thinks this is what that little boy needs, or from something else altogether?" Or simply, "How does that sound to the little boy?"

If the inspiration comes from a protector, rather than Self or from the Self of the target part, we help the protector relax back as usual. If the inspiration comes from the little boy, if the little boy says he wants the anointing, or if there is the sense that it comes from Self, we let it unfold and see where it leads. Profound spiritual experiences happen in just this way. If it seems to fall flat or go astray, we encourage consultees to hang in there and simply be curious with clients about why and what needs to happen next.

Some clients use the practices of their own tradition as an adjunct to IFS. They work with their parts in the sweat lodge, pray for or from a part, seek the benefit of ayahuasca ceremonies, or anything else. This is a client's right. More than that, the interplay of spiritual approaches often enhances and furthers the healing work. In these cases, consultants and consultees check themselves for personal notions regarding what should or shouldn't happen and then do their own work, as needed. Consultants teach therapists how to be helpfully curious with their clients about the interconnections between a particular faith practice and the client's IFS process. They can ask:

- How has (the practice) helped your process?
- How is (a particular target) part responding?
- How is your system responding?
- What needs to happen next?

Sometimes an altogether transcendent presence shows up. It appears in the form of light, a person who has died, angels, Jesus, Native American elders, spirit animals, a shaman, or just about anything else. Clients sometimes invite in presence to support the work; other times the appearance is spontaneous and not even necessarily from the client's own tradition. A first nation chief might show up for a Christian, Jesus for a Buddhist, angels for an atheist. Divine irony. But when it comes, however it presents, clients usually recognize its spiritual worth. They also feel vulnerable. Clients want to know if their clinician is comfortable with this kind of thing. They don't necessarily need you to believe in it, they just want to know if you can handle it – if they can trust you not to judge, dismiss, diminish, or otherwise imply in any way that they are "crazy." As consultants, we steady our consultees and help them accept these occurrences with calm and curiosity.

Most such manifestations come for the good – to lend energy or bring messages that contribute to the process. Sometimes clients report a malicious intent – what some have come to call *unattached burdens*. In-depth exploration of these manifestations lies beyond the scope of this chapter. Numerous IFS practitioners and healers have developed resources and reference materials pertaining to aspects of IFS and spirituality, including guides, unattached burdens, legacy burdens, and other topics. Consultants should familiarize themselves with these resources and know where their consultation clients can find them.

Self at the Core

"It happened again," Maria says, "and with a different client! This client had a religious part that felt responsible for saving everyone and all the other parts. The part said it felt like it was hanging on for dear life. I suggested that my client embody that part, and, literally, she was grasping upward to the heavens with her right hand. She felt her heart open toward this religious part and then there was a pulsating energy all around, and twinkly lights. She felt an arm come down along her right side and cradle her whole body. That part had been holding on, but now she wasn't … didn't have to: she was being held."

"How was that for you?" I asked.

"It was beautiful. And a little too easy. I felt like I should be doing something more to earn my pay. You know me," she smiles. "I did ask about unburdening – about anything that needed to be released or any message meant to be received, and tears started rolling down her face. 'I'm not evil, and I'm not an abomination,' she said. 'No matter what they say.'

"I had no idea that was in there!" Maria says. "It wasn't anything we had talked about. I don't even know if it was an unburdening or a message or what. I just know it made a difference. She looked lighter – and glowing. It changed how she feels toward her family. They didn't change. They still act the same, but what they say doesn't seem to bother her anymore, doesn't matter as much as it did. She even says she feels calmer around them and sometimes more loving. Whenever she starts to feel that need to grab again and hold on for dear life, she says she goes back to that sense of being held. Pretty amazing."

Pretty amazing, indeed.

When it comes to IFS, the nuts and bolts matter, the theory and the practice matter, but in the end, whether we are in the role of consultant, consultee, or client, or just out and about in our lives, a trusting relationship with Self lies at the core. At times Self-energy is apparent within the therapist-client relationship or within other human interconnections. We may sense Self on the inside as it manifests in a loving Self-to-part relationship. Other times we find it in nature, in the natural flow of the athlete, or in the creative impulse of the artist. As IFS consultants and clinicians, we simply follow the model, and we embrace the practice. Self shows up, and when it does, we are amazed and privileged to find ourselves, like Maria, included in the circle of someone else's grace.

Note

1 Case vignettes are fictionalized.

References

Butler Bass, D. (2018, June 26). #MeToo and the Spiritual Struggle for Gratitude [Blog Post]. *On Being*. [Based on Butler Bass, D. (2018). *Grateful: The transformative power of giving thanks*. HarperCollins]. Retrieved from https://onbeing.org/blog/diana-butler-bass-metoo-and-the-spirpitual-struggle-for-gratitude.

Longfellow, H. W. (1857). *Prose works of Henry Wadsworth Longfellow*. Volume 1. Ticknor and Fields. Retrieved from HathiTrust.

Minuchin, S., & Fishman, H. C. (1981). *Family therapy techniques*. Harvard University Press.

Schwartz, R. C. (n.d.). The larger self. *IFS Institute*. Retrieved from https://www.ifs-institute.com/resources/articles/larger-self.

Scorah, A (2020). *Leaving the witness: Exiting a religion and finding a life*. Penguin Books.

Sutherland, O. (2005). A family therapist's constructionist perspective on the therapeutic relationship. *Journal of Systemic Therapies*, *24*(2), 1–17. doi:10.1521/jsyt.2005.24.2.1.

Tervalon, M., & Murray-Garcia, J. (1998). Cultural humility versus cultural competence: A critical distinction in defining physician training outcomes in multicultural education. *Journal of Health Care for the Poor and Underserved*, *9*(2), 117–125.

11 Serving Those Who Served

Providing IFS-Informed Supervision and Consultation to Clinicians Treating Military Veterans

Sharon Cooper and Kimberly Corey

Introduction

Every July we train a new group of psychology interns fresh out of their graduate programs and eager to gain clinical experience in treating veterans. Some have family members who served in the military (a spouse, parent, or grandparent), some have served themselves, and some have completed training at another Veterans Health Administration (VA) hospital. Most, however, have little prior experience working with military veterans. The first step in orienting them to this population is to help them get comfortable identifying their own feelings about working with veterans, which is often a different approach than what they have experienced in graduate school. Most interns have been trained in cognitive behavioral therapy (CBT) and what is often called *third wave* (Hayes, 2004) evidence-based psychotherapies, such as acceptance and commitment therapy (ACT), dialectical behavioral therapy (DBT), and mindfulness-based cognitive therapy (MBCT). Given that few have any knowledge of IFS, what each new class of interns is rarely prepared for when they take our seminar, *Orientation to Military Culture*, is speaking for their own fears and concerns about working with this population. Over time, we have learned that most of them hear an inner critic that questions their competence or undermines their confidence in treating this population. This can be true for experienced clinicians as well when working with veterans who have complex trauma histories. We understand this experience very well, as we both started our own clinical training at a VA medical center almost 20 years ago. As part of our current clinical responsibilities, we supervise psychology interns who provide individual and group psychotherapy, consult with community clinicians who are working with veterans, and provide group consultation to clinicians at a local Vet Center.

Chapter Outline

This chapter explores the process of supervising and consulting with those who treat veterans who have served in the United States Armed Forces. We

DOI: 10.4324/9781003044864-11

describe strategies that can help supervisees, who may have difficulty building rapport given their civilian status, and underscore how common it is for therapists to have parts who collude with veterans who feel isolated, misunderstood, and alone once they return home. Through case examples, we illustrate the challenges many therapists face when their parts feel inadequate or helpless to support their clients given the magnitude of the losses they have experienced. In addition, we consider how to work with therapists' parts who can block Self-energy when the therapist feels overwhelmed by hearing detailed descriptions of physical and/or emotional trauma. We explore how to help consultees be Self-led when their own parts' political beliefs are in opposition to the war agenda, making it difficult to hold space for the veteran's parts who have harmed others in order to complete the mission and survive the brutality of war. Additionally, as supervisors and consultants, we discuss the important work of tracking and working with our own parts that may be triggered by the supervision/consultation process. Finally, we share IFS-informed strategies that support and assist clinicians to be "in the trenches" day after day while reassuring their parts that there is goodness and connection in the world. In this chapter, we use the term *supervision* when referring to unlicensed clinicians who we are responsible for training and who work under our license, and *consultation* when we are working with licensed independent practitioners who seek assistance in gaining clarity when they, or more accurately their parts, feel stuck in their work with a veteran. In addition, the case writeups in this chapter are based on compilations of our sessions rather than on direct transcriptions to ensure the privacy of our supervisees/consultees and their clients.

Military Culture

With its own language, beliefs, and traditions, veterans of the Armed Services have their own unique culture, which holds respect and honor as its core principles. Therefore, prior to working with military veterans, it is extremely useful to make a concerted effort to learn about military culture. Time invested in learning about the experiences of veterans will help the clinician more easily understand why certain parts in the veteran's system may have difficulty relaxing or assuming a new role once they return to civilian life. In our clinical practice, we have seen parts transform when provided with compassionate witnessing, and it has been our experience that updating parts of the system as to why it was important—even life-saving—that they did their job, helps extend compassion and appreciation to parts who often feel misunderstood and abandoned—not only by the veteran, but by their family and society at large. Taking the time to learn what it may have been like to walk in that veteran's boots, both during the time they were in the military and during their transition back to civilian life, will undoubtedly help build rapport and trust between therapist and client. Taking an interest in their culture is often seen as an extension of an olive-branch to those parts who believe that others outside of the military may not want to recognize that they needed to exist.

To address the fears and concerns of veterans' protective parts, we have found IFS-informed education to be time well spent. Similar to how a cognitive-behavioral therapist routinely provides education on the relationship between thoughts, feelings, and behaviors, IFS therapists can provide education that we all have parts, and that it is the work of our protectors (both managers and firefighters) to keep us safe from feeling overwhelmed by our exiled parts, who seek to be unburdened and healed. It can also be helpful to provide basic education on how veterans' parts, who took on extreme roles as a result of their military training in order to keep them safe, are different from the parts civilians rely on who have never served in the military.

Veterans are often relieved to understand that, when working with an IFS therapist, we honor all parts, even extreme ones, and that the goal is never to get rid of any parts, but to release them from the burdens they carry. Parts relax when it is clearly explained that it is our belief that they likely do not need to work so hard now that they are out of the military, and that they would benefit from getting a new updated role as they reintegrate into their civilian life. We also encourage consultees and supervisees to provide concrete examples to their veteran clients to further illustrate how their parts were influenced by military service. Learning that their inability to sleep is likely due to a "scanning part," who developed to protect themselves and others given that missions often occurred at night, can be a game changer. Helping them understand the positive intentions of parts can shift their thinking from fearing that something is fundamentally wrong with them to recognizing that they excelled at their job in the military. They are often relieved to learn that extreme parts can be updated and take on new, less burdened roles.

It has been our experience that providing IFS-informed education piques the veteran's curiosity about their own system and the interplay between their parts. They benefit from understanding that every part has positive intentions for them, even the parts that previously may have been villainized. It also makes our job as a "hope merchant" (Schwartz & Sweezy, 2020) easier, as we instill a burgeoning hope that under our watch, it is possible that they can create the civilian life they undoubtedly desire.

Building Rapport

Relationships can make the difference between successful reintegration to civilian life and feelings of failure and increased isolation. Veterans often say they feel closer to the people with whom they served than to their own family. Sometimes they state that the only time they feel "normal" is when they get together with their military buddies. This sense of disconnection from their families, their communities, and their own Self-energy can manifest in protective behaviors, such as avoidance and emotional numbing or even more extreme firefighter activity.

Relationship challenges often present in the therapy office as well, and a common question that trainees bring to supervision relates to building rapport. Veterans who may have experienced trauma are quick to lead with protective parts who feel highly misunderstood by others and feel isolated from their civilian counterparts. These protective parts are quick to verbalize that you can't understand what they have been through. They fear that opening up to you will further confirm this belief and create a greater sense of aloneness and isolation. These protective parts are often concerned that if they shared their story, we would reject them for their actions; alternatively, these protective parts may be polarized with other parts who are horrified by what they saw or did while deployed, and they may hate themselves and/or fear contaminating others with their stories. In response to this inner dynamic, veterans often shut down to protect others (and themselves) from the pain and internal confusion they feel, which contributes even more to feelings of isolation and a loss of connection to those around them.

In addition, many veterans have an idealized vision of their homecoming, only to be disappointed by their family's well-intentioned demands or lack of understanding. Family members may also harbor expectations of picking up exactly where they left off prior to the veteran's deployment, only to feel that they are living with a stranger. Spouses and parents are often ill-prepared to know how to make space for the veteran's parts who took on extreme roles while deployed. Many family members want the veteran to put their trauma "behind them" and "move on." The failure to adequately prepare families for what to expect when their loved ones come home translates into the veteran feeling unknown by the people who previously knew them the best; and if their own families can't understand them, many veterans think what chance does their newly assigned clinician have?

The challenges of building rapport with veterans are illustrated in the case of "Laura," who came for consultation when her client ended the session abruptly after she asked him if he wanted to work with the part who witnessed so much suffering on deployment. Laura came to consultation feeling stuck, not understanding why the Veteran angrily stated: "You weren't there. How can you even begin to understand me?"

Given what she learned about the challenges of reintegration to civilian life, consultation began with encouraging Laura to consider how this thought could be true for the part of the Veteran who may have attempted to share his story with family or friends without success. Laura noted that she did understand this was a manager-fear of the Veteran, but she felt somewhat frustrated as she had shared with him that she had experience treating veterans and even has veterans in her own family. In her mind, this disclosure should have been sufficient to demonstrate that she understands him and can be trusted. Consultation began with an exploration of the 6 Fs.

"Can you find the part in your body that is feeling frustrated with the Veteran for thinking you can't understand?"

"Yes, it's in my stomach and chest. It's a tightness, almost a slight pain."

"How do you feel toward this tightness in your stomach and chest?"

"I feel really irritated. I guess I'm frustrated with it too. I know it's not the Veteran's fault that he feels alienated, but what do I have to do to prove myself?"

"So, it sounds like one part of you understands how this Veteran may feel that no one can understand him, and another part of you is frustrated that you need to work so hard given how much personal and professional experience you have."

"Exactly! What do I have to do to show that I'm capable of helping him?"

"I wonder if the part who's frustrated would be willing to share more about its experience so that we can better understand what's happening."

With Laura's agreement and permission, the frustrated part was available and willing to tell her story. Through an exploration using the 6 Fs, we learned that the frustrated part was full of good intentions but often feared that her best efforts would not yield positive results. When asked to show the part it protected, a young exile appeared who held profound sadness at her inability to connect to her own father, who is also a military veteran. The exile showed Laura how hard she tried to please her father, who remained distant and guarded from his family due to his own protective parts that likely took on extreme roles during his military service. The exile had long-standing beliefs that, despite her best efforts, she would always feel unworthy of her father's love. After unburdening that part and having it take in the qualities of love, connection, and wholeness, the work felt complete, and Laura left the consultation session with clarity about how her own parts contributed to the challenge of creating a space for the Veteran to express his fears and concerns. She also gained clarity on her own pacing and why she felt compelled to work so hard to try and help veterans heal. In this case, consultation helped Laura explore her feelings and emotions, which led to a young exile from her own family of origin. Once unburdened, her system had greater access to Self-energy.

Inner Critics: Parts Who Challenge, Collude, and Polarize

Veterans are not the only ones who have parts who are skeptical about their ability to heal. Supervisees and consultees often present with fears that perhaps they aren't sufficiently skilled or talented to be able to help the veteran. Typically, when asked to share what is happening in the therapy room, most therapists describe hitting multiple roadblocks with clients who shut down, become irritable, or communicate that they are "too far gone" and beyond help.

Over time, we have learned from providing supervision and consultation with both new and seasoned clinicians that many of them hear an inner critic question their competence or undermine their confidence in treating this population. The inner critic might whisper to them: *What do you know about losing your best friend or waking up at night in a cold sweat screaming?* Younger clinicians might hear: *Don't tell them you were born after the Vietnam War and never heard of the Tet Offensive! Just nod and hope they don't ask if you know what that is.* Or they may hear an acronym they don't know, for example, IED, VBED, FOB, and think inwardly: *Do I ask what the acronym means, or will that undermine my credibility?* (See Table 11.1 for specialized terms).

For most therapists unfamiliar with this population, it's hard to be a confident hope merchant when they have parts who are unsure of whether they have the skills to help their veteran clients. In supervision and consultation, we teach clinicians that the job of the veterans' managers is to prevent them from feeling overwhelmed by the burdens they carry. Often that takes many forms. We help clinicians to not be surprised or flustered when they ask the veteran at the beginning of the session: "What would you like to focus on today?" and they get a response similar to "I don't know" or "You're the expert, you tell me!" or "I'm doing this for my wife. I don't really want to be here." Veterans' managers can also take other forms, either saying very little in therapy or talking non-stop about things that do not address their reason for coming to therapy, all of which have the intended consequence of preventing the therapist from getting anywhere near their emotional pain, shame, or guilt.

These experiences can cause a therapist to collude with the veterans' parts and "go with the flow," or polarize with the veterans' parts and get impatient. Such circumstances can also activate a caretaking part in the therapist, which prompts them to focus on case management needs in an attempt to

Table 11.1 Specialized Terms

FOB:
Forward Operating Base

IED:
Improvised Explosive Device

Tet Offensive:
In 1968 the North Vietnamese launched a series of coordinated attacks on more than 100 cities and outposts in South Vietnam.

VBED:
Vehicle Borne Explosive Device

Vet Center:
Community-based counseling centers that provide social and psychological services to veterans and active-duty service members and their families.

Veterans Health Administration (VA):
America's largest integrated health care system serving over 9 million veterans each year at 1,255 health care facilities.

contain their own sadness or helplessness. When therapists collude with veterans' parts, they may agree that they don't have the skills to help them and may wonder if this work is really for them. On more than one occasion, a supervisee has shared that they felt panic mid-session when one of their parts offered up loudly and clearly inside: *Wow, this guy really needs a therapist*, and then they remembered that *they* were, in fact, the therapist in the room tasked with the job of helping the veteran. Although this thought of wishing there were a more skilled therapist in the room often sparks laughter when brought to light in supervision, it is clear that there truly is a part within many therapists who often requires updating surrounding their proficiency in treating challenging cases.

Parts Who Feel Inadequate or Helpless Given the Magnitude of the Veteran's Losses

In supervision, we often work with therapists who are having difficulty accessing Self-energy due to having parts who feel overwhelmed. Sometimes therapists may be blended with younger parts of themselves who are not well-equipped to take a leading role in the therapy office. It is not uncommon for therapists' young, vulnerable parts to show up when faced with working with trauma clients, as young parts who are disconnected from Self-energy may get triggered by the stories they hear. These parts often want to help and may have a lifetime of experience soothing angry parts or helping to distract sad parts. However, these young parts, who were likely parentified in youth, can feel overwhelmed by the stories they hear and can overwhelm the therapist's system. If we can help these younger parts recognize that they have access to resources in the system that they did not have growing up, they will be able to release their role and allow the therapist's Self-energy to assist the veteran in unblending from their parts and accessing their own Self-energy.

When therapists are asked to identify their own roadblocks to success, they often describe parts who hold feelings of inadequacy or helplessness given the magnitude of the losses experienced by their client. Therapists report fears of pushing their clients too hard or asking them too much and triggering them to shut down or get angry. This is especially true when the veteran shares, "You're the first person I've ever told this to." Veterans often express fears that if they were to truly open up, they would be overwhelmed by their sadness and unable to function. Alternatively, veterans sometimes fear that if we saw the depth of their pain and the violence they witnessed or participated in, either we would be vicariously traumatized, or we would be horrified by their story and reject them. Therapists also worry that they may not be able to manage the potential outpouring of the veteran's emotions within the confines of the therapy hour if they assist the veteran in giving voice to the parts who hold these burdens. The following consultation with a therapist who works for an agency with a high veteran population illustrates this point.

"I just had a session this week that I don't feel good about."

"Can you say more about that?"

"I was really tired—the referrals keep coming in—and I think I 'phoned it in' a bit during the session; you know, went through the motions without being fully present."

"It sounds like that isn't your typical way of doing therapy."

"No, it's not. The Veteran's baseline is depressed and anxious, but he had been doing a little better recently. However, at this session, he started talking about a terrible nightmare he had the night before and how overwhelming his depression and anxiety have been this past week."

"How did you respond?"

"I'm embarrassed to say that I ignored his comments about his nightmare and overwhelming depression and anxiety and focused instead on what we can do to get him back on track. I think my 'cheerleader part' showed up. Instead of addressing the part of him that couldn't get out of bed, I focused on positive behavioral activation and concrete skills. It was like I forgot my IFS training."

"Are you aware of what your fears and concerns were in session about focusing on his depressive and anxious parts?"

"Given the intensity of his depression, my fear was that he would become so dysregulated that I wouldn't be able to complete our session in 45 minutes, and I had back-to-back clients all day."

"Hearing this, can you speak for your parts that showed up in session?"

"When he started talking about how depressed he was, and how horrible his nightmare was, I had parts that were saying: *OMG ... his depressed part is back again!* I felt frustrated initially, but as I think about it now, I think I felt sad and helpless."

"Can you tap into the parts of you that felt sad, helpless, and perhaps a little overwhelmed? What were their fears and concerns?"

"Those parts felt embarrassed because they thought I should be better than this."

"Does that part want to say more? Does it fear I will judge it?"

"I don't think you can judge me any more harshly than I'm judging myself."

"Would the part that judges you be willing to give you a little space so we can better understand what happened that day?"

"Yes, that part really likes consultation because it says: *We have to get our act together.*"

"Before we proceed, can you check to see if there are any other parts who may not be so on board with looking at this situation?"

"Hmm ... there is another part that is hesitant about looking at this issue. That's the part that feels overwhelmed and does fear you may judge me. It's afraid it will be ganged up on."

"Can you let the overwhelmed part know that our goal is not to gang up on it, but to help it not feel so overwhelmed? (Pause) How did it respond?"

"It liked that idea. That part is so tired."

"Would it be helpful to focus on the part of you that got overwhelmed in your session with the Veteran?"

"Yes, I think that would be really helpful. It was like this part of me forgot IFS, and I fell back on my CBT skills focusing on pleasant activities and behavioral activation."

"Would this part be willing to share with you a little more about how it has been feeling?"

"It's afraid that I've turned into a bad therapist. Between teleworking, Zoom meetings, social distancing, fears about contracting COVID-19, not seeing family and friends, it fears I have become less effective and have less energy for the work."

"It sounds like you have been working very hard trying to adjust to the current reality of living and working through the COVID-19 pandemic. And I hear that this part fears it has become less effective. Can you check to see if all parts feel that way?"

"Actually, most days I'm really proud of the work I do. I've been able to transition to telework without missing a beat, and most of the time I feel like I'm doing really good IFS work."

"Given that at times you feel very competent, and you do very good work, is there something about this particular client or his issue that made this part feel overwhelmed and caused it to focus on behavioral activation rather than focusing on the client's depressed part?"

"I'm not sure. This Veteran has had a lot of trauma, but I'm realizing how hopeless I feel about the work in general because this year has been so hard. There is so much suffering and the clients keep coming and coming, and I worry that they need more frequent sessions than I have available in my schedule. It makes me feel so tired and overwhelmed."

"Can you focus on the part of you that feels overwhelmed? Where do you feel it in or around your body?"

"There's a tightness, a constriction around my heart."

"Any fears or concerns about working with this part?"

"No. I know it needs my help."

"How are you feeling toward this part?"

"I'm curious."

"Can you ask that part if there's anything it would like to share about its experience that day?"

"It's saying that it wanted to focus on behavioral activation in session because it was afraid that I would get even more overwhelmed if we focused on his depression. It decided to flip into 'cheerleader/health coach' mode and focus on the benefits of exercise and social interaction as a way to improve his mood."

"After hearing that, how are you now feeling toward this part?"

"I definitely have more appreciation for that part because it really wants to help. This part wanted to help me coach him out of his depression so I wouldn't feel overwhelmed."

"Can you send this part appreciation?"

"Yes, it likes that. It's very proud of what it knows. This part feels like a health coach reminding veterans of all the healthy things they can do to feel better."

"Does this coach part know that you are a competent IFS therapist with a solid skillset?"

"Kind of, but it jumps in when the situation feels scary in order to protect me."

"What is its concern if it didn't jump in?"

"It fears that if we focused on the depressed part, it would get bigger and bigger, and the Veteran would want to stay in bed more and more."

"You said this coach part jumps in when it gets 'too scary.' Is it willing to show you the part it protects that gets scared?"

(Consultee tears up.) "Wow ... I just got this vision of being seven or eight years old. There was a time when my dad was depressed, and it was scary to see him that way."

"What did this young girl do when she saw her father depressed?"

"She sang or danced or tried to be charming to shift his mood."

"Did it help?"

"Yes, usually it helped, but it was stressful. She worried about her father a lot and wondered if she was doing enough."

"How do you feel toward her now?"

"I love her. She's the hardest working seven-year-old on the planet. She's amazing at reading the room. I realize now that she certainly doesn't know IFS, but she's great at recognizing when someone isn't well, and she tries to find ways to make them feel better. She accurately perceived that the Veteran wasn't doing well last session. I thought it was my exhaustion that made me 'phone it in,' but now I realize it was her."

"Does she know who you are?"

"Oh, yes. Since my Level 1 training, I have done some work with her. We love each other; but that day, for that session, I didn't show up, she did. She's letting me know that she went to the session by herself."

"Can you update the little girl and show her the part of you that is a confident and competent IFS therapist with skills to handle these situations?"

"Yes, I want her to know that she doesn't have to be the therapist and do my job."

"How is she reacting?"

"She got so excited. She wants to go on Spring Break!"

"Ask if there is anything else that she needs from you?"

"No, she's okay now. I'm letting her know that she can play and doesn't have to come to session anymore."

"How do you feel now?"

"I feel *so* relieved. And I feel like I have a lot of clarity."

"Were the other parts, like 'the health coach,' watching?"

"Yes, they were surprised about the whole thing. The health coach still recommends that I get more sleep, which I appreciate. He's letting me know that if I sleep more and get more rest, my little girl can play more and not feel like she needs to run the show."

"Sounds like good advice. Can you focus back on your chest and see how you're now feeling?"

"There's no tightness. I don't feel that constriction anymore."

"Before we end, focus your attention on that depressed Veteran and see how you are feeling toward him now."

"I feel completely different. I feel able to befriend his depressed part and work to understand his fears and concerns. Right now, I have no dread, no hesitation. I want to get to know that part of him that doesn't want to get out of bed."

Therapist Parts Who Block Self-Energy

Listening to stories in which people were ordered to kill enemy combatants or tortured people to get information or went on a search and rescue mission after an IED explosion only to find bloody remains, can be painful for the veteran to share with their therapist because it awakens in them both the horror of the event as well as their own survivor guilt. Given the graphic nature of these traumas, it is therefore understandable that during session both veterans and therapists may have parts that get activated and block their Self-energy in an attempt to manage their own emotional response.

Veterans will sometimes share stories to prove to you that they are "broken" beyond repair and that there is nothing the therapist can do to help them. Sometimes they will refuse to share a story to "protect" the therapist from suffering in the way that they still suffer from these painful memories. And sometimes a part will share the story with the hope that we can somehow help them make sense of it. Further complicating the presentation, many veterans have complex trauma dating back to childhood. In every case, hearing the realities of war or the intensity of the trauma can evoke parts in the therapist that block Self-energy.

When listening compassionately to the veteran's story, sometimes parts come up in the therapist which they may not be aware of initially. The therapist may notice that they are confused as to where to start or concerned that this veteran is in an unhealthy relationship and doesn't have the external supports in place to make the changes necessary to heal, or perhaps they are engaged in extreme firefighter behaviors (heavy alcohol and/or drug use, frequent episodes of road rage, recent suicide attempt, brushes with the law, gambling away their whole disability check, or engaging in intimate partner violence). Therapists can have parts that get scared if the veteran is thinking about self-harm or engaging in high-risk behaviors, fearing that their best efforts to unburden the underlying trauma will be thwarted or not done in time to prevent serious self-injury. It is easy during these times for therapists' parts to polarize with these extreme firefighters and insist that the veteran create a safety plan without engaging in the necessary work to befriend these extreme parts and understand their fears and concerns.

There are also therapist parts that collude with the veteran's hopeless parts and feel that, no matter what they do, the veteran cannot sustain the gains they make, whether in improved mood, ability to work, or engagement with family. Sometimes the veteran's hopeless parts may take the form of despair, and no matter how much the veteran seems to improve in the therapist's presence, they return the next session in what appears to be the exact same emotional place. It's as if their depression is like a rubber band that expands and gives the therapist and veteran hope in the moment, only to spring back to its baseline of despair the following session, causing the veteran's and therapist's hopeful parts to feel deflated, believing that change is not possible. It is at these times when consultation can be invaluable. When months or years of therapy seem to yield little movement and the therapist realizes that they are either colluding or polarizing with the veteran, it is important for the therapist to work with their parts that are likely blocking connection to Self-energy.

When A Therapist's Political Beliefs are in Opposition to the War Agenda

"I lost my moral compass the moment I walked off the plane in Vietnam," the Veteran told his therapist, who sought consultation on this case. The consultee shared that this Veteran referred to himself as a "monster," and he had witnessed interrogations at gunpoint, blamed himself for his fellow Marines being killed in an ambush, and took part in the burning of villages. He also described how angry and confused he felt when he returned home in uniform and was confronted by angry protestors. The therapist shared that her efforts to provide psychoeducation to her client were not helping him heal, despite the fact that he appeared to understand that infantrymen are asked to do things in combat that they would never do in civilian life. Despite her reassurances, he insisted that he was "going to Hell." No matter how hard she tried to challenge his thinking and remind him that he did these acts when he was 18 years old and has been a very loving and caring husband and father since then, he held strong to his belief that God could never forgive him for what he witnessed and for what he did. She said he had been carrying this pain for over 50 years. After getting some background information and acknowledging how hard she had been working with this client, we were able to focus on her fears and concerns.

The therapist began, "It's really hard watching him suffer. I guess I feel helpless, and at the same time, I'm ashamed to admit that part of me really hates what he did."

"Can you say more?"

"I'm ashamed that I was someone who protested the Vietnam War. I could have been someone who called him a 'baby killer' or held signs calling him a murderer."

"Sounds like you're both carrying shame, for different reasons. Would you like to get to know this part of you a little better?"

"I would, but I'm afraid it will negatively impact my work with him."

"What are your concerns?"

"What if I learn that he actually killed unarmed women and children? What if, instead of feeling compassion, I find his actions reprehensible?"

"And if you learned that what you fear was true, what would be your fears and concerns?"

"That I couldn't work with him any longer."

"And if that came to pass, do you have a colleague you think would be willing to work with him, or would you be willing to refer him to the VA or a local Vet Center?"

"I never thought of doing that. I would be okay with that."

"If you could get to understand this shame so it didn't interfere with your work, would you be interested?"

"Of course."

"Are you available to hear from the part of you that holds shame for protesting the Vietnam War?"

"I am. I can see what I was wearing the day we marched on the Washington Mall."

"How old were you?"

"I was 18 years old and a freshman in college."

"So, you were the same age as your client."

"Hmm, I never thought about that."

"Can you ask that 18-year-old student what inspired her to join the march on Washington, D.C. to protest the Vietnam War?"

"She said we were trying to stop the deaths of thousands of American troops and Vietnamese civilians."

"How do you feel toward her hearing that?"

"I have a lot of compassion for her. It took a lot of courage to do that."

"Can you send her that compassion? (Pause) How is she responding?"

"She turned toward me."

"Does she know who you are?"

"No."

"Can you tell her who you are? (Pause) How is she responding?"

"She's crying and hugging me."

"Is she interested in learning more about your life since that time?"

"Yes!"

"Go ahead and update her." (Longer pause) "How is she responding?"

(Chuckling) "She's surprised I became a therapist."

"Ask her if she didn't have to carry the identity of a Vietnam anti-war protestor and could unburden the shame she has carried since that time, would she be interested?"

"Absolutely!"

We then did the healing steps of IFS to unburden the parts of her that were carrying both anger toward the government and shame for directing her anger at the individual servicemen who were drafted or volunteered for the Vietnam War.

"How are you doing?"

"I feel a lot lighter."

"Are you willing to see yourself in your office with this Veteran?"

"I am."

"How are you now feeling toward him?"

"I have a lot of compassion for him. He volunteered to go to Vietnam in place of another Marine who was married and just had a child. That was a very selfless act. And he has been trying to redeem himself by helping others and donating money to children's charities even though he doesn't have a lot of money."

"Do you think you can still work with him?"

"Absolutely."

Tracking Consultant Parts

Although we recognize that there are many ways in which parts may get activated, we find that there are two common ways therapists respond to clients when the therapist is triggered and having difficulty accessing Self-energy. They often collude with their clients' parts, or they polarize with their clients' parts. The same can happen in supervision and consultation. Sometimes we find ourselves engaging in caretaking or cheerleading of our supervisees to encourage them along the way, and sometimes we polarize with them feeling frustrated that, despite supervision, we see the same patterns repeating themselves. The IFS model teaches us how to track and attend to our parts in order to access more Self-energy. We will highlight just three common parts that have shown up for us when doing this work.

Caretaking Parts

Caretaking parts can often show up when our supervisees present with their vulnerable, overwhelmed parts, triggering in us a desire to ease their discomfort. Unfortunately, caretaking parts often masquerade as Self-energy. Caretaking parts differ from Self-energy in that they have a clear agenda and often can take on burdens that are not theirs to carry. This can present as a preoccupation with the supervisee's well-being, providing unnecessary reassurance and reducing their workload in order to make the supervisee's job less burdensome. These caretaking parts may be further reinforced if the supervisee expresses appreciation for our assistance and guidance. As supervisors, caretaking parts can derail us from our training mission, which is to prepare supervisees to be competent therapists and to recognize and manage their own parts that show up in the therapy office. When providing supervision or consultation, it is important to bring Self-energy to our caretaking parts to reassure them that we don't need to carry other therapists' burdens.

Analyzing Parts

In supervision or consultation, there is often a lot of information presented at the beginning of session in a reporting type of style, with little-to-no information about what the therapist was experiencing during the session. As consultants, we sometimes notice ourselves thinking, *Oh this is a tough case.* Often our "analyzer part" is trying, cognitively, to figure out the underlying dynamic between the parts. When we notice that we are focused on solving the "puzzle" of the consultee's case, we are likely blended with an analytical part. If we can ask that analyzer part to give us some space, which affords us the opportunity to bring in more Self-energy, we can better serve our consultee by asking, "How do you feel when you are in the room with the client?" or "Where do you feel stuck?"

Teaching Parts

Consultants have the luxury of listening to a consultee's case without being "in the trenches" themselves. At times we may feel tempted to short circuit the process and provide psychoeducation about the parts we believe are activated in both the consultee and their client, rather than use the IFS model to help the therapist more deeply explore the parts of themselves that may be impacting the therapy process. Although there are times when psychoeducation may be very relevant and effective, in general, if we can get our own "teaching" or "expert" parts to give us some space, it is often more helpful to explore where the consultee feels stuck in session.

Connection to Self-Energy is Essential to Sustain Hope

According to Simionato and Simpson (2018, p. 1431), "[b]urnout is a leading cause of work-related problems for psychotherapists, their clients, and the profession of psychotherapy." How, then, do clinicians remain "in the trenches" day after day and still reassure their parts that there is goodness and connection in the world? How can we continue to be hope merchants when our job is to witness the suffering of humanity? The answers to these perennial questions are both universal and personal.

Self-to-Part Connection

The universal answer is that we need to continue to connect with our own Self-energy. Our parts need to be shown that our system will feel more replenished when connected to Self-energy, and one of the best ways to do this is to do our own work to help our parts heal. By doing our own work, we will be more available to those we serve. The more we can access our own Self-energy, the less activated our parts will become, and the faster our clients' parts will trust us.

The personal answer is that we need to find meaningful self-care activities that help reconnect us to our Self-energy. Complementary and integrative practices may help relax our body and mind (e.g., massage, yoga, tai chi); connection to community may help nurture our heart, re-invigorate our mind, and reconnect us with our spirit (e.g., consultation, spending time with friends, staying connected to the IFS community), and Self-affirming practices may help us feel directly connected to Self and Spirit (e.g., meditation, prayer, sacred music, yogic breathing).

Additionally, we cannot overestimate the value of humor, play, and creative pursuits to reduce burnout and allow our parts that hold pain to release their burdens. As IFS-trained clinicians who have witnessed many exile/protector unburdenings, the number one desire of the unencumbered exile is to play. Connection to our younger parts and asking them about their need for play can quickly reunite us with Self-energy and reduce burnout and compassion fatigue. Creativity is one of the 8 Cs, and it is an inner resource that is always available to us. In diligently serving others and helping their parts connect to Self-energy, we must not forget the importance of connecting with our own Self-energy.

Conclusion

When providing supervision or consultation to those who treat military veterans, IFS provides us with a framework to understand the invisible war that often exists within the veteran long after they return home and put on civilian clothes. The beauty of the IFS model is its simplicity and its universality. Regardless of our personal histories, we all share a common humanity and benefit when our parts connect to Self-energy. With IFS-informed supervision and consultation, we can improve the care veterans receive by compassionately addressing the parts of the therapist that may unintentionally block healing. By doing our own work and being open to the supervision/consultation process, we will be more available to those we serve. The IFS model of psychotherapy allows us to truly welcome home the veteran, not just to their family, but to their own Self-energy.

References

Hayes, S. C. (2004). Acceptance and commitment therapy, relational frame theory, and the third wave of behavioral and cognitive therapies. *Behavior therapy, 35*(4), 639–665. doi:10.1016/S0005-7894(04)80013-3.

Schwartz, R. C., & Sweezy, M. (2020). *Internal Family Systems therapy* (2nd ed.). The Guilford Press.

Simionato G. K., & Simpson, S. (2018). Personal risk factors associated with burnout among psychotherapists: A systematic review of the literature. *Journal of clinical psychology, 74*(9), 1431–1456. doi:10.1002/jclp.22615.

12 Consultation with Therapists Who Have a Serious Illness

Roberta Rachel Omin

Introduction

When therapists discover they have a serious illness, it is at their discretion whether or not to enter consultation or raise this in an existing consultation relationship. If and when the therapist's ill health is raised, consultants may not be comfortable and confident helping the consultee navigate the choppy waters facing them in their clinical work. Some therapists use their personal therapy to help their parts concerned about the illness, though this may not necessarily address their professional practice. In this chapter, I share some of my personal story – how I came to specialize in consulting with therapists who find their personal and professional lives upended by illness. I also include data based on extensive interviews with over 100 therapists and clients. While most clients conveyed that they would prefer to be told honestly about their therapist's illness, the actual practice of self-disclosing on the part of therapists was often uneven, inconsistent, and ambivalent. I suggest that Self-led disclosure is in the best interests of both therapist and client and include a roadmap of how this might be done. Two clinical examples in which I consult with therapists around their illness are included, together with another in which I incorporate consultation into a therapy relationship with a seriously ill therapist.

My Story: How My Specialty Came About

When I was diagnosed with breast cancer 12 years ago, I shared my experience with some oncology mental health colleagues with the intention of learning how to navigate my personal journey. Some came forward privately in supportive yet hushed tones while disclosing they had also had breast cancer. Some became my breast cancer mentors. It took months before I received a clear diagnosis and more months with two lumpectomies before I had a mastectomy. I was in my own therapy at the time, working with my parts terrified and threatened about having cancer, since both my sister and mother had had breast cancer. I asked my seasoned therapist, "Do I need to tell my clients? I wonder if they can tell something is off with me.

DOI: 10.4324/9781003044864-12

What should I say about taking time off for medical appointments?" She replied, "Clients won't notice. They are involved with themselves." I recall not finding that fully believable but did not question it. She did not check in with me at any point about these concerns. In my practice consultation, I shared my situation, but again my clients were my primary focus – not whether and how my medical issues might be impacting my practice. Eventually I told my clients I was having minor surgery and would be off for a few days. Afterwards, two clients unexpectedly asked how the "minor surgery" had gone. I braced and paused to gather myself. "I have early-stage breast cancer and had a lumpectomy, which has hopefully removed all the cancer," I said. On my own, each step of the way, I was figuring out what to say and when to say it.

Ten months into my journey, I had a mastectomy and began chemotherapy. As I was preparing to lose my hair, I experienced a nagging "crisis of authenticity." I felt like a phony, wondering how I could wear a wig to cover up my "condition" when my clients were implicitly relying on me to be trustworthy and authentic. What kind of example would I be setting by trying to "hide" something that I suspected was having an impact in the room whether I acknowledged it or not? Such an obvious cover-up felt very wrong. My crisis of authenticity had not surfaced earlier in such a pressing way, and it had certainly not been nudged out in either my therapy or consultation. My "working hard" parts were in the lead, as one client was later able to tell me.

Organically, I had to become ready to open up about my medical circumstances, yet I still lacked clarity about how to do that. I shared my dilemma with two colleague friends, who offered a simple and clear solution, "Tell your clients: 'I have early-stage breast cancer. My prognosis is very good. I will be having gentle chemo to be sure the cancer is all gone and will be wearing scarves when my hair falls out. Do you have any questions?'"

This became my introductory script. From there, conversations with clients were individualized based on what they brought up over time. It only took a few minutes of their sessions.

My hardworking parts relaxed, my concerns that rescheduling clients for medical appointments would ruffle their feathers ceased, and when I was not at my best toward the end of chemotherapy, I was able to own that. Most clients were compassionate, expressing concern that what they were going through was not as important as what I was going through. I assured them their lives were important to me *and* they continued to do their work, including following their trailheads arising from my self-disclosure. I became Self-led, authentic, calm, clear, and more present.

My curiosity deepened both about what other therapists did in similar circumstances to mine and about their clients. I developed several questionnaires along with an interview request that was put on clinical listservs. The doors opened. Many therapists and clients came forward. I interviewed therapists with different cancers at various stages as well as heart disease, strokes, multiple sclerosis (MS), Lyme disease, Parkinson's, need for surgery, sudden hearing loss, diabetes, and amyotrophic lateral sclerosis (ALS). Their experiences ran the gamut from single acute events to chronic diseases, including progressive and terminal illnesses. I spoke with clients whose therapists had these illnesses, some of whom had died. Colleagues shared a range of experiences with peers who had either not revealed their illnesses to their clients or had revealed their illness but worked until they died and never consciously ended the relationship. It was quite revealing. Over 100 people shared their stories. Some had been more Self-led than others. A meaningful body of information evolved. (The existing literature was sparse.) I began leading workshops on the topic. Ellen Ziskind, a colleague, believed in the importance of this work. Her immense support and editing skills enabled me to publish an article in the *Psychotherapy Networker*: "To Reveal or Not to Reveal: When the Therapist Has a Serious Illness" (Omin, 2020). Clinicians continue to contact me to tell me their stories and ask for consultation.

Illness Impacts Us All

No one is immune from frailty and mortality. When the therapist's personal life is interrupted with illness or injury, working with our parts is necessary for our well-being. We are challenged and devastated with the gamut of extreme emotions/parts, such as shock, fear, helplessness, hopelessness, anger, sadness, shame, terror, and vulnerability. This life-changing experience creates a "before," "during," and "after." Our valued assumptions are challenged. We are altered in the process. We require time, attention, curiosity, and self-compassion to process and work with our own trailheads before we can become grounded enough and even consider Self-led disclosure with colleagues and clients.

Therapists' Parts Have Something to Say about Illness and Work

Therapists I interviewed shared the following explanations, beliefs, and fears of their parts as to why they had not said anything about their illness to their clients and colleagues:

- "The illness was too much to handle personally, without bringing my clients into it."
- "Therapy is about the client, not about the therapist."
- "I needed to keep my referrals and income, so I didn't share this with colleagues."
- "I needed to feel hopeful, that I would lick this, and did not want to have to deal with clients worrying about me."

- "I couldn't face telling. I was overwhelmed, scared, and afraid of falling apart."
- "I didn't want to appear weak, dependent, or vulnerable with my clients."
- "My therapy practice was a refuge away from my illness."
- "If my clients knew how sick I was, they'd have left me."
- "I am the healer, a caretaker, a giver – I can't be the one in need."
- "I felt ashamed of being ill, about the part of my body affected."
- "It's my fault. I brought this on myself."
- "I can't bear to think about not working or no longer existing one day."

Why Self-Disclosure Matters

When illness interrupts a therapist's life, an energetic experience is alive, however muted, within the therapy room. Yet, we've been taught not to talk about ourselves, except for the benefit of our clients. I believe it is in the best interests of clients that therapists disclose, rather than hide, when serious illness has struck or mortality approaches (Omin, 2020). Many clients have relational traumas and attachment injuries due to previous abandonments, secrets, and betrayals. Their hypervigilant parts, so necessary to their survival, pick up implicit cues that something is amiss. Doesn't it stand to reason that the way we handle our illness in the therapeutic relationship can activate clients' previous woundings?

Therapists may imagine that their illness will go unnoticed. However, we cannot know which clients will pick up on what cues. Even if a therapist shows no obvious symptoms, something implicit in the energy field is not being talked about. If changes are visible and either denied or not talked about, there is an elephant in the room. Both therapist and client feel it. The client may feel betrayed when they discover the illness was *intentionally* withheld. If the practice abruptly closes, or there is no farewell at all, they likely will feel abandoned. Client interviews show that when a therapist stops practicing without an ending and a shared farewell, harmful repercussions ensue. Clients are left on their own to face the rupture and attachment breach, complicating their grief.

How Specialized Consultation Can Help

The growing edge for us as therapists is when the personal and professional intersect. If we wish to disclose with access to enough Self-energy, we may need to do our personal work first, including following trailheads we might otherwise not have followed. We can help our clients face that we are human beings with medical vulnerabilities. In turn, our Self-led disclosure provides clients an opportunity to follow their own trailheads to previous attachment wounds and exiles. Therapy may be enhanced, not derailed. On the other hand, if disclosure is dominated by the therapist's situation or needs, then it is parts-led and may be detrimental. In my interviews, it was clear that clients wanted to know – to be told by their therapist of their illness or impending death. They did not need to know details. They expressed gratitude at "being included." Self-disclosing provides an opportunity for shared resiliency. Clients benefit from a meaningful, corrective, and healing experience of honesty and authenticity (Omin, 2020). And it may help prepare the client for possible eventualities. Contextual truth is always better than falsehoods, sidetracking, or omission. Processing together the impact on the client speaks to the health and safety in the relationship.

A Roadmap is Needed

For the consultant of the ill therapist, an accompanying roadmap can be useful at such a time. Therapists frequently utilize IFS consultation with the intention to come into Self-leadership by working with the professional and personal parts that impact or blindside their clinical work. During this specialized consultation, the consultant encourages the therapist's curiosity and compassion for parts that are impacted by the illness. Unblending enables the therapist to have a Self to "illness parts" relationship, making room to unburden and heal wounds. More Self is then available in the therapy room, which is of particular importance when working with clients who have attachment wounds and trauma histories. Accessing core therapeutic values, such as integrity, courage, and authenticity, and co-creating safety and trust, consultant and consultee can explore options so Self-led choices can be made. Some of those choices are about whether to remain silent or self-disclose, how to proceed from there, and how to assess the impact of those decisions so that no harm or the least possible harm is done. Each therapist who becomes seriously ill faces these pressing choices. If their condition is terminal, the time to process and come into "enough Self" will not be optimal, may be considerably abbreviated, and might necessitate emergency consultations.

For those who decide to reveal their health status to clients, I have developed the following Principles of Contextual Self-Led Disclosure. These guidelines are relational, non-linear, and reflect an evolving process rooted in the therapist:

- having a critical mass of Self-Energy;
- reflecting on their own attachment style(s) and how this impacts their beliefs and values regarding the therapy relationship;
- holding in awareness the client's core themes, attachment style(s), and wounds; and
- attuning to the impact of the self-disclosure and the illness, or impending mortality, on the client–therapist relationship.

Principles of Contextual Self-Led Disclosure

Access Self-Leadership and Self-Energy

First and foremost, help Self come to the fore. This includes being curious toward:

- parts that hold beliefs and feelings about uncertainty, vulnerability, intimacy, dying, and death;
- protectors aligned with the position: "Don't self-disclose";
- polarized protectors who sense some benefits to be had in disclosing;
- parts that say "Do self-disclose" to meet their needs of being cared for by clients;
- parts who may hold cultural burdens or biases, such as "therapists don't get sick" and "caretakers' needs come last";
- parts who may hold professional burdens or biases, such as "good therapists don't talk about themselves" and "I must protect my clients from negative experiences/suffering"; and
- exiles impacted by your illness, treatment, and prognosis.

Access increased Self-leadership by:

- being kind, compassionate, and patient with yourself;
- enlisting support from your family, friends, trusted colleagues, consultant, and own therapist;
- giving yourself time to process your own trailheads and metabolize, so that you can make Self-led choices about when, how, and what to disclose.

Pre-Disclosure: Prepare for Contact with Clients

Reflect on your attachment style(s) and how it might impact clients. How do you hold your clients and the relationship?

- Identify your core clinical values around self-disclosing: trust, safety, being authentic, honesty, integrity, courage, modeling managing life's difficulties and challenges, etc.
- Remind yourself of each client's attachment wounds, trauma history, and core needs in order to put the needs of each client at the center.
- Decide what and how much you want to disclose, which may vary with each client.
- Ask yourself what each client might need for a healthy and positive continuation of your relationship.
- Give yourself permission to set limits and boundaries relationally.

Self-Led Disclosure with Clients

Don't wait to the end of session – this may be more than a one-session conversation.

- Speak with simplicity and honesty about your illness.
- Reflecting your core values, share why you are disclosing as it relates to your work together, i.e., the impact on your client based on their history, your availability, possible leave of absence, disruptions in treatment.
- Ask client what they understand.
- Give client permission to ask questions as well as share feelings and concerns. If you need to think about a concern, assure client you will get back to him/her/them.
- Notice what your client wants to know and does not want to know. Explore any ambivalence about knowing. Support client's protective system.
- Respect your own process, boundaries, and timing (you don't have to tell all clients at once).
- Remember: You have the prerogative to not answer certain questions. Explicit privacy is not secrecy.

(Return back to the first section on therapist Self-leadership to check on how parts are doing, seek support.)

Following Up on Self-Led Disclosure

- Be curious toward clients: "What is my illness bringing up for you?" "Do you have any concerns or questions?" You are giving the message that "You can talk about anything" and "All parts are welcome in the here and now with me."
- What comes up for clients are trailheads for continued vertical (intrapersonal) therapeutic work.
- What comes up in the relationship are trailheads for horizontal (interpersonal) therapeutic work.
- If clients seem to be holding back, you can gently ask about what cannot be spoken – this gives parts permission to share.
- "Unmentionables" may still be held back, such as, "Will you die and abandon me?" "Will I get my needs met?" "Am I a burden?" or "I'm scared."
- Together you may need to discuss whether temporary or permanent transfer to another therapist would be appropriate for your client.
- Some clients may not be able to stay in therapy because of their history or circumstances. Help them speak for parts so they can leave with Self-energy.

- Be aware of pitfalls and ruptures and make repairs with clients where you can.
- Notice your own capacity to make good decisions.
- If you are no longer able to work effectively, a termination process needs to be implemented, including referral to a trusted colleague, saying a mutual goodbye, acknowledging growths, and anything that is significant between you both.
- Prepare a professional will (your professional body will have resources; see Pope & Vasquez, 2016).

(Return back to the first section on therapist Self-leadership to check on how parts are doing; seek support.)

Michael

Michael is a 60-year-old IFS therapist diagnosed two years ago with multiple sclerosis (MS), a chronic, progressive disease that leads to increasing disability. Michael's symptoms had been barely noticeable, so he didn't think seriously about sharing his illness with clients until his gait was less steady and he fatigued more. He had read my article in the *Psychotherapy Networker* and contacted me, "Because it made me rethink how I'm dealing with it." We had a few phone consultations. Michael was seeing about 30 clients weekly. His support network was strong, including his wife, adult daughters, close friends, as well as an excellent team of doctors. Over time he had revealed his illness to his extended family, friends, and suitemates. He felt supported, loved, and more authentic in sharing his news rather than keeping a secret that would be outed later as his body would inevitably decline. As his diagnosis became more real to him, there were a lot of tears. Michael had done a great deal of inner work before he even contacted me. He stated calmly, "I can shape how I want to live this part of my life, what meaning I'm giving it. It took me time to come to this – it was not an overnight acceptance."

During our initial consultation, Michael realized he needed to go through a similar, yet different, process with his clients. I asked him, "What did you discover about yourself in revealing with your friends and suitemates?" He shared, "I had to be ready!" I wondered what that meant for him.

Michael explained, "I had parts that weren't ready to accept the reality of this illness. I had to come to terms with it within myself, with solitary time. As well, I needed time to process it with those very close to me. I needed to mourn that my life was forever changed, for the life I'd hoped to have, for what this would mean for my wife and family and for me as a professional, a breadwinner, and a full human being."

Knowing MS would progress to a debilitating illness, Michael came to realize how grateful he was for what he did have in his life now. He needed new dreams. "This is a spiritual reckoning. We create the life we want even when it isn't any longer the life that we'd imagined." Clearly Michael had done much internal work with his parts about his illness. I shared how touched I was with his deep courage and authenticity.

I was curious, "What do your parts need as you contemplate revealing this illness with your clients?" Michael acknowledged he needed to be as Self-led and centered as possible. He knew that sharing would be a process for his clients as well as for him. He also intuitively knew that the conversation would be ongoing as his disease would be changing over time. We both took a deep breath and paused.

Michael explained, "Some clients have noticed changes. I shuffle a bit, and there's a cane by my desk. Some noticed I seem more tired and have asked about my health. I had not been quite ready to reveal what was already in the room until I read your article. There is something synchronistic about this." He continued, "If I were my client, I would be curious about my therapist." I suggested that would be a good place to start – with their curiosity.

"What would that mean for how you are with your clients?" I asked.

He replied readily, "I want to speak with them in a real way, answer their questions, while at the same time not overwhelm my system or theirs. It will be an emotional and physiological challenge for me. As I've discovered with my previous conversations, I can handle them one at a time. I expect each one will be different depending upon who the client is, and our relationship."

I agreed. I suggested that he think about who needs to know sooner rather than later – to triage his disclosure. Michael sighed – that had landed well.

Michael voiced a part that wanted to avoid talking in person to protect himself from being too vulnerable. He considered writing a thoughtful and inviting email, while another part didn't want to short-change his clients by not communicating in person. Another part experienced a sense of urgency, "I don't even know how my body will be different next week if I have a flare up. It's a scary journey!"

Michael expressed concern about a client he'd worked with for 30 years, for whom he'd been an anchor. In the session following his disclosure, she had looked online about his illness. She spoke of her "love" for him, knowing that eventually his illness would be life-changing. "I saw this conversation as her gift to me and to herself – to feel her love. I was willing to have this difficult conversation with her, even though a part of me was dreading it precisely because of her attachment to me. We courageously learned how to have our hearts open with each other."

This client was healing an attachment injury in the moment through the meaning of their relationship. She felt she was being let in and received – that she was considered, seen, and taken seriously when he said, "You can handle this." Her family did not handle anything. Michael reflected, "I honored her history and our relationship history. This is the beginning of a longer conversation which we will come back to. In a certain way, I'm doing the best work I've ever done." Facing his vulnerability, he was more inclusive of his needs and being with himself.

Michael is working with Self-leadership on multiple levels – living with self-acceptance, self-compassion, his personal life meaning, and his spirituality. His illness parts are unblended, they are a part of him and not equated with all of him. "I'm managing my practice, being deliberate, disclosing in manageable doses and not more than I can handle. My self-critical parts don't get caught up with things like changing session times. I change them more easily because I need to. As part of my self-care, I'm learning to pace my energy. Male clients ask if it's okay to hug me. Some ask if I will be retiring."

Michael continues to have courageous conversations with his clients.

Professional Wills

Because Michael intends to work for as long as possible, I brought up the issue of having a professional will. Most people have parts that avoid doing their personal wills because those parts don't want to confront the inevitability of dying. It's understandable that parts also deny the need for a professional will, which would put provisions in place should the therapist become incapacitated or die suddenly. My experience has been that not having a professional will is also a phenomenon of protection. Therapists living with an illness need support to get to know parts that avoid having a professional will with an invitation to another outcome. As consultants, we are in a unique position to bring our Self-energy to this conversation.

Provisions of a professional will might include:

- An emergency response leader or team to notify clients in a timely and sensitive manner about the therapist's circumstances.
- A clear way to access therapist's calendar, client contact list, and records.
- A pre-arranged plan detailing how clients would be notified and what would be said, giving consideration to the impact on the client getting this news and with the intention of supporting (and not harming) clients.
- A list of referring therapists or an assigned replacement.
- In the event of death, an invitation to a memorial service for clients to have a way to mourn their special relationship.

Michael saw creating his professional will as an essential and necessary coverage for his clients – as an act of love. Based on our consultations, I believe Michael's onward journey with himself and his clients will hold the same integrity, thoughtfulness, and compassion that he has already demonstrated.

Sandy

The Initial Consultation

Sandy, not IFS trained, was diagnosed with early-stage breast cancer. She had read my article, "To Reveal or Not to Reveal: When the Therapist Has a Serious Illness," and reached out for a consultation in how to continue in her full-time practice as a trauma specialist while dealing with her illness.

At our first online meeting, I explained that in this kind of consultation I have found it best to pay attention to the personal aspects of one's life as well as the professional. The context of who she is, what her resources and supports are, and what all of her has to say about her "illness" experience is just as important as how to work with her clients. In our consultation sessions, we shuttled between her personal life and her professional life.

Sandy, a 45-year-old woman, had done an inventory with her family and friends – who could give her emotional support and who would help on a practical level. At the end of the consultation, she expressed concerns about finances, changes in her appearance, and how she could get her own needs met. Naming these deeper fears was extremely important.

"Surgery is in two weeks. The medical piece is squared away. I'm very clear about my decision to have a lumpectomy," she told me. She knew that post-surgical treatment would be based on the biopsies and tumor markers.

Second Consultation Session Pre-Disclosure

"Are there parts of you saying, 'I don't want to disclose my medical issues to my clients?'" I asked Sandy.

"Yes, I worry it will be more than I want to deal with. Part of me is concerned it will activate their attachment issues which will then play out. They might use the information the wrong way."

I asked her specifically what she was concerned about, and I acknowledged, "Any of that could happen. I can help you with this."

"I'm aware of the potential harm for my clients if I don't disclose. It could be injurious to their safety and trust. Using your article, I've begun thinking about how to do that. I've got this script drafted: 'I have some uncomfortable news. I was diagnosed with early-stage breast cancer – it is treatable. I hope you will feel free to talk to me about your reactions. We will also need to work out what you can tolerate in terms of disruption to our appointments, and whether I can meet your needs.'"

"That sounds clear and succinct. When do you think you will tell your clients?" I prompted.

"Not at the end of the session so there is some time for them to speak for how they are initially impacted."

Consultation Session Post-Disclosure

Most clients thanked Sandy for telling them, responding with warmth, kindness, and surprise. They were touched that she revealed her news. They wanted to keep working with her and were fine if she had to take time off.

The client Sandy was most concerned about cried and said she didn't feel she had a right to her feelings and that she couldn't verbalize them yet. In response to my curiosity about the client's attachment injury, Sandy explained "She fears I'll die, and the loss would be too much for her. She needs information from me and to be reassured." As we talked about the ways to shape the continuing conversation with this client, Sandy visibly relaxed. We held awareness of this client's attachment wounding while helping Sandy feel she could still maintain her boundary about what she was and was not okay disclosing. The aim was to meet her client's needs as well as her own. Being aware of her inner comfort zone was her right and her self-responsibility, while sharing what her client needed to know for her own safety. Sandy sensed that this way of sharing could be beneficial for the treatment and their relationship. Once Sandy had this frame, she felt confident she could take it from there. In their next session, the client exclaimed, "I knew you would leave me. I can't trust you." We had anticipated this reaction, and although at first Sandy believed she had done the wrong thing, she recalled my suggestion and asked the client, "What would it have been like for you if I had not trusted you enough to tell you?" Sandy and I expected this could be a trailhead for further work together on trust. Sandy became clearer about the importance of helping clients understand their reactions to her medical situation as their own trailheads for therapeutic work. It didn't have to become about her.

Another client Sandy had been working with for ten years had a cooler response, stating, "I'll find another therapist and then we can wrap it up." With her hand on her heart, Sandy told me, "It was jarring, like I was replaceable." The client's avoidant attachment style was evident in this exchange. I explained that such clients were likely speaking from protective "I'll replace you" parts and with "I'll abandon you before you abandon me" covering their wounds of "I don't matter." This resonated for Sandy. She was able to reassure each client that she could continue to be present for them while going through her own treatment.

A third client with historical and current trauma concerned Sandy, "I don't want to add to her feelings of insecurity in the world. I don't want this safe relationship to be the source of uncertainty or shakiness." However, Sandy was clear that truth telling was the foundation of a secure attachment and hiding the truth was not an option. She saw the necessity of explaining to this client why she was disclosing, that it was for the client's safety and trust to know up front from her rather than risk hearing something later from somebody else. With Self-energy, Sandy communicated her caring, sensitivity, and open acknowledgement of her client's life struggles along with regret that issues in her own life might be echoes of past painful relationships in the client's own.

Therapist's Self-Leadership and Self-Energy

Sandy used the Principles of Contextual Self-Led Disclosure as a guide to the process and as part of the ongoing therapeutic dialogue. She wanted to know more about Self-energy. To her it meant the core authentic personhood. She realized that her wellness had been a gift that she feared losing. Then a part took over, believing "now I am a sick person, I am not grounded, not stable, and I am inauthentic." I wondered if she could rephrase this as "I am a person with an illness." This landed well.

Sandy was burdened with the belief that she needed to be "strong, solid, and steady, presenting my professional parent side to my clients." She also worried that her emotions could eclipse her clients' needs and interfere with being empathic. "I present as polished, in control, appropriately warm and caring. I can pull it together as if I am confident about the situation." I called these "parts" of her.

Sandy also conveyed a great sense of being burdened by her family, "While they support me, I am supporting them." I listened compassionately as Sandy explained her protective system, referring to her "caretaker parts." She recognized she leads from these parts with her clients. Sandy took a deep "aha" breath, signifying a new clarity, an organic, unblending space between the protectors and how they can run her life. I offered, "Self is aware of these parts and how hard they are working for you. While those parts have a really good intention for your system, they can also interfere with your true ability to be present for yourself and for your clients. There is a difference between caretaking and caring."

Sandy got it in the moment, both of us knowing we could spend time with these caretaker parts if we continued to work together. For now, she had an appreciation of how they played a significant part in her life and prevented her from being her more authentic core Self.

Gaining Insight though the Experience

Sandy shared some insights she had gained about herself as a therapist. She had come to view herself as human, vulnerable, and more complex. She had felt polarized responsibilities – to help clients process how disclosing her medical issues affected them while also wanting to maintain a safe, stable environment, which, to parts of her, meant not self-disclosing. "I wanted to do no harm, be the safety and stability for my clients. Now I realize my trauma-informed style was too rigid and heroic."

I added that the therapist's existential health crisis, while potentially traumatic for the client, is also different than the client's childhood trauma. For the client, the triggering of exiles by the therapist's self-disclosure of illness provides an opportunity for those exiles to be witnessed and healed within the therapeutic relationship if that is something the client wishes. Therapist self-disclosure need not trigger a re-enactment of earlier trauma history. Rather, the health crisis can open the door wider to the client's inner vertical therapeutic work, while the horizontal relational work between therapist and client can provide a reparative attachment experience. Sandy was appreciating these distinctions.

The previous case studies illustrate how, when sought out, IFS consultation can work well for both IFS-trained and non-IFS-trained therapists. A further opportunity for specialized consultation also arises when therapists enter treatment due to a serious illness or develop a serious illness during the course of therapy. I believe it is possible to shuttle between the roles of therapist and consultant by asking for and being given permission to put on our consultant's hat alongside our role as therapist.

Tim

The following case study illustrates how and why I, as therapist, shuttled to the consultant role, as needed, while holding my therapist self at the same time. My relationship with Tim demonstrates how hard it is, at times, to access Self-energy under the pressure of serious illness and impending death.

Tim, a therapist with some IFS training, sought me out for psychotherapy because he knew I worked with therapists dealing with serious illnesses. He'd been coping on his own with advancing lung cancer for five years. He had no regular consultation arrangements in place and chose not to get this support. Tim's life was fraught with the ongoing traumatic stress of new metastases, frequent medical crises, and treatment changes. He was often anxious, painfully aware that he would eventually die from the disease.

It wasn't until Tim was to be away from his practice for eight weeks following another surgery that I asked for and was given permission to put on my consultant's hat. I was curious how he planned to handle his absence with his clients. We welcomed and appreciated the parts that did not want to self-disclose. "Therapy is about the client; I don't want to scare them away. I need to maintain my professional identity." I offered to do a "mini workshop" with him right there in the session, introducing him to how to have a conversation based on the Principles of Contextual Self-Led Disclosure. Tim appeared genuinely open and receptive.

The next week he reported, "I did it, I informed my clients that I had some cancer that needed to be removed. I got that out of the way." He had checked that item off his list. "No one asked me any questions, and I didn't want them to." I could feel a part in my chest tighten. The mini workshop hadn't had the intended effect. I realized I had been influenced by a part with an agenda, telling myself the story that Tim's clients would suspect something was very wrong that he wasn't telling them, and that he needed to. Having done some of my own U-turn, I asked Tim, "Did you have parts that didn't want to talk about your illness with your clients but went along with it for me?" He nodded. Tim had a part who wanted to please me by disclosing that was polarized with a part who feared telling. Tim and I spent some time making a repair. Going forward, welcoming parts with objections to self-disclosing, even if out of his awareness at the time, had to be on my radar.

A few months later, Tim needed to have immediate brain surgery. He wasn't capable of contacting his clients, and a colleague stepped in to do that for him. After surgery, Tim returned to work prematurely. He was having some difficulty expressing himself because of where the brain tumor had been. A pushing and overriding manager part of him was in charge, and my parts were concerned about his lack of self-care in returning to his practice so quickly.

Tim hadn't shown interest in what his clients had been told about his sudden absence. He hadn't thought to have a conversation with his clients upon his return to work. A critical part of me was stunned by Tim's lack of curiosity and poor judgment. Another part was aligned with and protective of his clients. I identified with them as not mattering enough for Tim to be curious about how they were impacted by his abrupt departure. After I helped my parts unblend, Self could hold the bigger picture – Tim's brain was affected, his executive functioning likely compromised, his protective system was in extreme survival mode, and his remaining time might be short.

I remained Tim's therapist/consultant and tried to manage my parts. At one point, Tim alluded to the possibility of selling his practice sometime in the future. I struggled with my judgmental parts wondering, "What if Tim doesn't end with his clients in a relational way?" My parts wished for the right questions to help Tim go deeper and be more curious.

Tim shared his feelings around the unfairness of dying in mid-life. "Should I retire?" was polarized with his terror of "giving up." I was present with his fears and his questions. Despite constant extreme fatigue, Tim continued to work. He gave me permission, as both his therapist and consultant, to challenge him. "I'm concerned about you," I said. "Your body needs time to recuperate from the chemo. What if you took a temporary leave of absence from your practice, took the pressure off, and rested your body from having to show up in all the ways you do?" This would offer him some respite. We checked in with both of his polarized parts. They liked the suggested compromise, which was neither giving up nor retiring. We worked on an email to his clients about his leave of absence and an expected date of return. He offered the name of a covering therapist for those clients who needed it. He sent it out right away.

In the first weeks of his leave, Tim looked much better. He had more energy and was present in his body. The weight of the world had been lifted from his working and caretaking parts. He spoke for his sadness regarding not wanting to give up his practice and his identity as a clinician. Reaching out to his friends, he started to actively receive support – a crucial shift for him, as he had defined his life as being a giver, not a receiver. For Tim's next oncology appointment, a close friend accompanied him to help ask questions. Tim was relieved. His oncologist was not giving up on him even though he would not answer, "How long do I have?" Furthermore, Tim was responding well to a revised, less toxic chemo regime. His cancer markers came down dramatically.

A month before Tim's expected return to his practice, he announced to me that he had resumed seeing clients. I was surprised at what I perceived to be his impulsivity. This part had shown up before. I was curious, "What did your clients ask you when you returned?" He acknowledged, "They wanted to know how I was. I played it down and talked about them." Talking about his illness in a relational way with his clients was more than his system and his attachment style could handle. His protectors were more persistently in the lead again. Implicit direct access with compassion, curiosity, and presence from my Self to Tim's parts was the primary therapeutic approach.

This challenging case is a reminder to therapists (and consultants) that however well-intentioned and skilled, when living with a serious illness that threatens their life, a therapist's stalwart protectors may not feel safe enough to trust Self to lead. Also, the impact of the medical processes on the human organism may prevent the capacity to do in-depth work. All this may inhibit having a 'good enough' relational farewell ending, leaving what may be unfinished and unresolved for the therapist as well as for their clients.

In Closing

When a therapist's life and body are threatened by serious illness and impending death, the personal and the professional collide. Therapist parts can feel thrust into an abyss of uncertainty, vulnerability, chaos, and overwhelm. This, when combined with absences for medical appointments and treatments, poses challenges for their professional life, and in particular, their relationship with their clients. Clients come to therapy with their hopes and dreams, their traumas and attachment injuries. Therapists may also have attachment injuries and pre-existing traumas, therefore, specialized consultation and/or personal therapy are likely to be beneficial.

Consultants need courageous and compassionate Self-energy to hold the space for all their consultees' parts in this human and humbling experience and to make repair where parts take the lead. As consultants accompanying therapists faced with serious illness and possible death, I hope you are inspired by my story and the case studies.

As therapists, I hope you are encouraged to reflect on what sort of support and challenge you would want and need from a therapist or consultant in such circumstances. The theory and practice of Internal Family Systems therapy along with the Principles of Contextual Self-Led Disclosure provide an in-depth framework from which to draw.

References

Omin, R. R. (2020). To reveal or not to reveal: When the therapist has a serious illness. *Psychotherapy Networker, 44*(1), 40–45.

Pope, K. S., & Vasquez, M. J. T. (2016). *Ethics in psychotherapy and counseling: A practical guide* (5th ed.). Wiley.

13 IFS Consultation

Fostering the Self-Led Therapist

Fran Booth

Practitioners of Internal Family Systems understand the systemic complexity that occurs when two people sit down for a therapeutic conversation – a seemingly simple act. Successful therapeutic interventions rely on astute awareness of who is talking to whom among the internal multitudes. The ideal leader for therapeutic conversations – the state of compassion and curiosity, known as Self-energy – can be hidden or buried amidst the tangle of multitudes. The IFS practitioner seeks to cultivate recognition of these various states in clients and themselves; one aim of therapy, and therefore of consultation, is to accurately assess which of the various internal multitudes may be guiding a therapeutic conversation in any given moment.

Like many psychotherapeutic models, IFS posits it is important to explore the therapist's reactions to client material, noting they can serve as helpful partners in the therapeutic process, providing important insights into our clients' struggles. At other times, activated parts in the therapist can derail the therapeutic conversation, causing the therapist to lose the capacity to maintain a clear focus on the client's process, to understand what is occurring, to know what is needed and how to respond to the client calmly and compassionately. When activation occurs, it is considered a *trailhead* – an invitation to turn inward, toward parts that may need attention and healing. Trailheads and U-turns (Schwartz, 1995) challenge the therapist to take responsibility for personal parts that interfere with therapeutic conversations. IFS consultation assists with the skillful discernment between internal activation that enhances understanding the client and distinguishing therapist's parts that interfere with effective therapeutic connection and thoughtful clinical interventions.

IFS Consultation

Many models focus on the therapist's clinical presentation of the client as a starting point for consultation: personal and developmental history, precipitating events, family factors, culture, race, current stressors, external constraints, etc. In IFS, this information is embedded in a comprehensive, contextual, and broadly inclusive understanding of a client's parts. The parts themselves hold the history, the story, the events, the impact of race and culture, etc.

DOI: 10.4324/9781003044864-13

Some models of supervision and consultation maintain a focus on the healing of the client; the personal material of the supervisee is noted but not necessarily deemed essential. The IFS consultant seeks to foster growth and healing for both therapist and client. Often the IFS consultation contract is limited to simply identifying and unblending activated therapist's parts; the assumption is that the therapist will engage in therapy, as needed, independent of consultation. However, an IFS consultation contract can include permission to follow trailheads through all the IFS steps of healing. Together the consultant and therapist differentiate those trailheads that deserve attending to in personal therapy and those that can benefit from efficient, targeted therapeutic attention in consultation. Additionally, the IFS consultant serves as a parts detector for multiple systems (consultant, therapist, and client) and integrates awareness of the larger societal, cultural, and global environments within which these systems operate.

Ingredients for successful consultation relationships are analogous to qualities present in successful therapeutic relationships. These include, the importance of trust, the feeling of being understood, the respectful holding of vulnerability, and the sense that help and guidance are available.

This Chapter

The acceptance and normalization of the multitudes within has contributed to the recognition that therapist parts can and do, at times, interfere with Self-energy leading therapeutic conversations. This chapter presents a consultation case study of a therapist addressing and healing activated parts that interfered with maintaining a Self-led connection with her clients.[1] Consultation supports the exploration of activated parts to determine "what belongs to whom," and assists with the U-turn, unblending and healing activated parts. This chapter also highlights a relational repair process involving acknowledgment, accountability, and the self-disclosure of therapist parts to support and deepen an authentic therapeutic relationship.

The reader will note the application of several IFS processes, including unblending, unburdening, legacy unburdening, age update, and direct access with an exile. Other sources offer more descriptive details for these interventions (Schwartz & Sweezy, 2020).

This chapter uses the terms *client, therapist*, and *consultant*, while recognizing that practitioners, healers, coaches, lawyers, educators, healthcare providers, and many others may also benefit from U-turns, trailhead investigations, and acknowledging their parts with others. The clinical case material features two White, cisgender female, heterosexual clinicians; the hope is that the concepts presented will enjoy wider application.

Join Us in the Consultation Room

Jane, a talented and experienced IFS therapist, has been consulting with me for several months. With the aid of advanced trainings and previous consultation, she embodies the IFS protocols. She has done personal work in other settings; she demonstrates significant self-awareness and insight. In general, she proficiently identifies and unblends her parts and returns to clinical Self-leadership. However, as you will see, for a period of time, consultation focused on short-term, targeted therapeutic work to attend to activated personal parts.

Jane begins our regular consultation meeting with the declaration: "I want to transfer this case."

I, Fran, immediately notice the intensity of Jane's experience; I calmly take a deep breath to deepen my capacity to be present to all of it. I want her to know and feel she is not alone with her feelings. "I am right here with you. Tell me more."

Jane begins to tell me more. "I have started seeing this client since we last met. She begins every session with an outburst of feelings. It's like a dam bursts open, and her frustration and discouragement pour out. She speaks fast, with lots of energy. Her family and friends are ridiculous and insensitive. They don't care. They're selfish. She is furious at them. Then, every so often, she suddenly collapses into total helplessness. She cries, 'What's wrong with me?' Soon she's back to rapid-fire talking, venting about her pathetic life." Jane sighs and looks down.

"Yes. I get it. How about we start by trying to sort out what you are experiencing?"

Jane sits quietly for a moment. "Sure."

"Imagine you are sitting with her. Notice what you are experiencing."

"I feel so frustrated. This client is so hard to work with. There's actually a part in me that feels a lot of empathy for her family and friends. I think to myself that this client's anger and helplessness must be really hard for them to take. She complains that they leave her, but I feel she pushes people away."

"I understand. And what happens inside of you as you're noticing all of this?"

"I want to pull away from her." Jane moves her upper torso away and sighs. "And that makes me feel awful. I just don't think I can help her. I'm not helping her." Jane sighs again. "Maybe somebody else could do a better job." Jane slumps in her chair. "I am trying to stay present, but internally, I'm not there. I feel pretty helpless. I'm always thinking that there's more I should be doing. But I don't know what it is. I know that my wanting to pull away from her signals a problem." Jane sighs, drops her head lower and is silent.

"I get this. Something here is hard for you. Is this all of what you wanted to tell me?"

"Yeah."

"First, I want to acknowledge how important it is, and how helpful it is, that you are so aware of all that you are feeling. And that you can tell me all of it. See if you can let this truth sink in for a moment."

"I know that's true."

"Good. I know we can figure this out together. This is unusual for you – to feel so overwhelmed."

Jane nods. "Yeah."

"Let's pause for a moment. Can you bring some attention to what you are feeling?"

Jane pauses and turns her attention inward; she relaxes, a bit. "That's a little better."

"Great. Shall we return to your client for a moment?"

"Sure."

"Can you see the parts cycle? Your client expresses anger at her family and friends, then feels helpless, and then self-critical. She spins from protector to an exile, to a critical protector. We both know that this type of intensity often occurs for clients with a traumatic history."

"Oh, right." Her shoulders soften.

"Your body relaxed. What shifted for you?"

"Well, first, paying attention inside helped me settle some. And what you said makes so much sense to me: the parts cycle."

"Good. What are you understanding now?"

"I get it. All that rage … it's a protector part. A part that's in a protest."

"Yes."

Jane's clarity is emerging. "And now I can see that it protects a vulnerable exile who likely feels alone. It shows up as helpless and overwhelmed."

"Yes."

"And then the critic, 'What is wrong with me?'"

"Yes."

"Calming down and seeing the parts cycle, helps a lot. I have a sense of what to do next."

"Good. What's next?"

"Maybe some direct access with the anger or with the helplessness or maybe with the whole cycle of parts."

"Yes!"

In our remaining consultation time, Jane imagines herself back in the office. She sees her client in her mind's eye and initiates a role-play to practice "speaking" to her client, "I see how intense this is for you. These feelings are so strong. And they move fast. I sense how overwhelming this feels. We can figure this out. Let's be with these fast-moving parts together."

Reflection

Jane began our consultation meeting struggling with her client's hyperaroused cycle of parts. Because Jane is an experienced therapist, I hypothesized that the difficulty was not in her knowledge base, but in her reactions to the clinical presentation. Her client's intense parts cycle activates parts in Jane carrying frustration and helplessness. I sensed and saw the tension and frustration in Jane's body. I heard it in her tone of voice and in her pressured speech; I saw it in her facial expression. I knew her feelings deserved attention. I noted the frustration and helplessness in the client and the co-occurring frustration and helplessness in Jane. I settled myself and invited Jane to notice the impact of this client on herself. As she did this, more Self-energy became available; her parts relaxed. She remembered what she knows – to "parts detect," to "see" the cycle of parts. She knew her next steps.

Although she regained her clinical acumen, I was curious about this strong reaction in Jane. This level of distress often signals unresolved childhood wounds impacting clinical work. Since Jane's consultation contract includes permission to explore trailheads and heal her wounds, I relaxed, gently held my reflection, trusting that when the time became right we would address any blocks to clinical effectiveness.

Jane's U-Turn

In our next meeting, Jane gives a quick update on the client presented previously. Although still struggling, she feels less overwhelmed and is able to help her client map the cycle of parts. She brings a different relationship to consultation today: "I have a different case for today. I'm so frustrated. This client feels hopeless. She is expecting me to help. It feels urgent, and I feel overwhelmed and stuck."

"I get it. Anything else?"

"I'm feeling … 'I don't know how to do this. I can't help.' I get confused. And I get frozen."

"Is it okay for us to explore this? Shall we start here, with these thoughts and feelings?"

"Yup." She smiles a bit sheepishly. "It feels familiar."

"Yes." Jane seems aware of the similarity with the earlier consultation exploration.

"Let's explore this cluster of parts together. Take a moment and see what is there."

As I extend this invitation, I quietly take a deep breath to settle my system, quickly scan for information from my parts, and return my focus to Jane's experience.

Jane pauses for a moment. "Someone, something inside is saying, 'It's too much work being a therapist. It's too much responsibility. I can't do it. It's too much pressure.'"

She looks at me and sighs. "My client is stuck. I'm stuck."

"Notice where in your body you experience this."

"It's in my chest and belly. It's subtle right now."

"How are you feeling toward the sensations?"

"Interested."

"Great. Stay a bit."

"There's an image now. I'm six years old. I am with my mom. She's in bed. She is depressed."

"Okay to go to that little girl?" I hypothesize that we may be in the scene at the root of Jane's triggered feelings. My question implicitly asks protectors for permission to be there.

"Yes."

"Great. Be with her."

"She's relieved I'm here. But she's feeling overwhelmed. And frozen."

"How do you feel toward her now?"

"Interested in her. She's checking me out. I am there with her. She wants me to feel it, to join her, know her."

"Are you okay with that?" I check to verify that Jane's Self-energy is leading this process.

"Yes."

"So, feel what she wants you to know. Stay with her until you sense she feels known."

We are quiet while this occurs.

I notice that my breath is rhythmic and spacious, my attention is focused on Jane and this girl. I have a picture in my mind's eye of a six-year-old girl.

"She is relaxing." Jane's shoulders soften and drop a bit.

"Great. See if there is more she wants you to know."

"She feels so overwhelmed. It's all too much."

"If that makes sense to you, let her know."

"Yes."

"Does she sense you get it?"

Jane nods. Again, there are a few moments of silence. "She's looking at me. I think she's beginning to trust me."

"Great. Stay with her checking you out, 'till she comes to trust you are here with her." Again, I quickly scan my body and focus of attention; I notice I feel relaxed, engaged, and drawn into this moment. There is silence as Jane is focused internally.

"She is closer to me now."

"Good."

Reflection

Many contemporary psychotherapeutic paradigms posit unprocessed trauma is held in the body (Van der Kolk, 2014). When Jane turned toward the sensations in her body, an image of her younger self immediately emerged. I wondered if we had met the part of Jane that felt overwhelmed by her client. After obtaining explicit permission, I invited Jane to connect with her younger self. This young girl is standing at the bedside of her depressed mom; she feels helpless, overwhelmed, and frozen.

From previous meetings, I knew that Jane's mother had suffered and become incapacitated by a major depression when Jane was six years old. As the eldest, young Jane helped with meals and childcare for three siblings. As Jane connected with her younger self, she learned and understood what she needs now and what was needed at the time, which was someone to help her be with feeling overwhelmed and helpless as she experienced her mother's depression. Jane offered her younger self compassion; I did, too.

Releasing a Legacy Burden

As Jane continues to be with her young part, it becomes clear that in addition to the weight of helplessness the young girl feels, she also carries some of her mother's emotional pain – a legacy burden.

We return to Jane and her younger self. Jane begins, "She feels my care for her."

"Good. Ask her to see if she is carrying anything that is not hers."

"She's carrying Mom's shame. Shame about being sick, shame about being stuck."

"Oh. That makes sense, doesn't it?"

Jane nods.

"Let her know it makes sense to you."

"She appreciates that. A lot."

"Let her know that she is not meant to carry Mom's shame. We can help her with that. Would she like help with that?"

"Yes."

I invite Jane to give her younger self permission to no longer carry her mother's shame. We begin the IFS process originally taught to me by Michi Rose called "legacy unburdening," which is designed to release burdens, such as negative beliefs or feelings of shame, depression, fear, or despair, that have been passed down from previous generations (Sinko, 2017).

As is common, we discover fears that inhibit Jane's younger self from immediately letting go of her mother's shame. If Jane gives back the shame that does not belong to her, will there be anything left to her? I coach Jane to reassure her child that we understand she has been carrying this shame for so long it feels like the core of her identity; however, she is much more than this burden of shame. Young Jane slowly ponders this idea; she is intrigued by the possibility this could be true.

Jane's inner six-year-old has another concern. If she releases the shame she has been carrying with her mother, will they still have a connection? Like all young children, this child wants and needs her bond with her mother. Sharing her mother's shame has been a way to be connected. We remind her that once the burden of shame has been released, she and her mother will find new ways to be connected. Again, the truth of this makes intuitive sense to young Jane. Now she can, and does, release the shame that belonged to her mother.

Although, at the end of the session, I am aware that young Jane still carries considerable emotional pain. We agree to pause for now and to continue this work in our next meeting.

Reflection

As Jane shifted her attention from the girl back to the office and to me, she acknowledged this part blends with her in sessions with this client and others. She recognized the importance of giving this part attention. (Her cognitive parts returned, bringing another layer of integration.) I had valued being present in this process; I had felt privileged to be there for Jane and her young self. As the work had unfolded the pace of my breath had slowed, my heart had opened. The "space" between us and the "space" inside Jane had resonated with interconnectedness. As Daniel Siegel writes:

> When we feel Presence in others, we feel that spaciousness of our being received by them. And when we reside in Presence in ourselves, others, and indeed the whole world, are welcomed into our being.
>
> (Siegel, 2007, p. 160)

Meeting Jane's Protectors

Jane began our next meeting reporting that during the week she was aware of her younger self waiting in the background of her consciousness. Each morning she took a few quiet moments to reassure her of the intention to return to her soon.

"I can sense her now," Jane begins.

"How are you feeling toward her?"

"Hmmm. I just spaced out and I can feel a constriction in my chest."

"Oh. I wonder if there are parts that want to shut down connecting with her? Check to see if that's so."

"Yep. They don't want the little girl to get overwhelmed."

"Okay. That makes sense. I bet, in the past, they saw her get overwhelmed. No wonder they are concerned. Let them know it makes sense they are concerned."

"They are listening."

"Let them know, we don't want her to be overwhelmed either."

"They heard you say that. They're relieved."

"How do you feel toward the 'spacing out' part and the 'constriction' now?"

"Interested."

"Great. Be with them."

"There's less intensity now."

"Good. Invite them to share anything they want to you to know."

"They're showing me just how they helped."

"Yes. Let them know, you know they helped." I notice I also genuinely feel that these protectors did and do help. "How do you feel toward them now?"

"Appreciative."

"Let them know. ... What's that like for them, to take in your appreciation?"

"They're relaxing, even more."

"Great, ask them how old they think you are?"

"Six-years-old."

"Oh. Let them know how old you are today." Jane shares her current age.

"What's that like for them?"

"They are surprised."

"That makes sense. Invite them to keep noticing you are older now."

"They are taking that in more. They are still not sure they can trust me to help."

"That makes sense. Stay with them until you sense they trust you more."

Reflection

Jane began our meeting ready to continue the work with her younger self. Initially, we met two protectors worried that the young child's feelings would overwhelm her, as had occurred in the past. I coached Jane to validate the protectors' concerns. We agreed that we did not want Jane's system to be overwhelmed. As Jane validated these concerns, the internal intensity diminished. I invited Jane to inform the protectors there is more help available now; Jane shared her present-day chronological age. In IFS, an "age update" is a specific intervention addressing the tendency of traumatized parts to "freeze" at the age of a traumatic event and to be unaware that time and life have continued. And from that experience in the past, these parts continued to influence present-day thoughts, feelings, beliefs, and behaviors. Also, these young, wounded parts were so accustomed to managing alone, they initially did not notice more help was currently available. Once Jane's protectors sensed the possibility of help, they relaxed; Jane connected with her six-year-old self again.

Unburdening Jane's Exile

"The girl is here now with me."

"Great. Be with her. Just as she is. Notice if she knows you are there with her."

Silence.

"She is relaxing with me."

"Great. Stay until you sense your connection with her is solid."

"She is looking at me. She is happy I am here with her."

"See what else she wants you to know."

"I'm getting an image. I'm six years old. The church has handed out compassion boxes with pictures of starving kids. I didn't know there were starving kids in the world. I'm horrified. Starving children in the world … why isn't anyone paying attention to this? Why isn't anyone helping?"

"Jane, let her know you want to know all about this. Notice if she knows you are there."

"No, I'm very blended". Jane knows she is no longer with her younger self.

"May I talk to her?"

"Sure."

"Great."

"Okay. So, you're the young girl inside Jane! First of all, I want to tell you, I'm so glad you're here. Thank you for talking to me directly. I've gotten to know you a little through Jane, and I'd like to know you a bit more."

"Okay."

"I know you are six years old. I know you have some big worries about starving children in the world. I heard and felt you when you said you were horrified when you learned about starving children. I can only imagine. Do I have this right?" Jane nods.

"I did hear you ask, why isn't anyone paying attention to this? That is a very important question. I am glad you asked it. Something about this situation you find yourself in does not seem right. Am I getting this?"

Letting her child part speak, "Yes."

"Can you tell me a bit more?"

Jane's child continues to speak, "All these children need help, and no one is doing anything about it!"

"Yes. You see that, and that troubles you. Tell me more."

"I feel like I'm trying to help. And I'm trying to get help. No one comes."

"Oh, wow. You are trying to help, and you want help, too! Of course, you want someone to come. Wanting to help and wanting to get help make sense."

I continue to speak directly with this young girl inside Jane; my vocal tone and pace of speech communicate caring and acknowledgment of this painful experience. She shares more of her experience of trying to get help, to no avail. When my relationship with the girl feels solid, I move to have Jane join us, with her Self-energy in the lead.

I begin making the invitation, "This is a wild idea, but what if there was more help inside that could come and be with you, right now? Would that interest you?"

"Hmmm … Yes."

"You could try this. If you soften your feelings, even a little bit, you could have company inside. You don't have to change your feelings at all, just make room for Jane, who is here too. Then you will not feel so alone with these worries and feelings. Would you like to try this?"

"Yes."

"So, let it happen. Soften your feelings and allow Jane to be with you now. You can tell her, too, about your efforts to help the starving children. You are trying to help. And that you want help, but no one comes."

After a moment of silence, "Jane, are you there with her now?"

"Yes." Jane's Self is now available to be with the overwhelmed child inside her.

"Great. Be with her. Let her know all that you heard and understood."

Jane repeats to her young child what she has heard and learned while I was speaking to the girl. As the girl shares more with Jane, she remembers how completely overwhelmed and immobilized she felt by her mother's sadness. She remembers desperately wanting to help and intensely wanting and needing more support. She wonders, why wasn't there more help? Jane acknowledges the feelings of helplessness and aloneness; she stays with the six-year-old until she feels fully understood. Giving company to her younger self helps; the healing begins. Together they complete the IFS ritual of unburdening; they release the aloneness and helplessness that had been hidden for years.

Reflection

In the face of her mother's depression, young Jane was filled with help-lessness and aloneness. These feelings were overwhelming; she displaced some of her emotional distress onto starving children. As you read, the experience of overwhelm occurred again in the present; just as it had tran-spired in childhood when Jane needed more help.

When these feelings limited Jane's capacity to be with her younger self, I shifted and spoke directly to this young child – in IFS terms, direct access with an exile. I stayed in that process until the child felt held, understood, validated. Then the intensity of the feelings naturally softened, and Jane's Self-energy was available again to be with the child. Undoing early alone-ness is crucial to healing trauma; young Jane is now able to integrate that which had been previously overwhelming.

Healing the Protector, "I Must Help"

Jane begins our next meeting reporting that she continued to track parts that emerged with clients. I notice Jane's greater ability to observe her parts and not be taken over by them. Jane has more Self-energy available, both when with her clients and in the recounting to me.

"I no longer feel frozen in the session with clients. I have more energy available. But I am noticing other parts are still getting triggered by the client I presented previously. I have a part that continues to feel responsible. It believes it is my job to look after her and clients like her."

"So, you have more energy and are less frozen, great. And you are noticing a part that feels very responsible."

"I do feel responsible. I am her therapist. So many other therapists have failed. She is in so much pain. So many relationships have ended. Her life is so lonely. She has no friends. I notice that I can get caught problem-solving. I hear from this part of me that believes I must help."

"Okay. Good awareness! It sounds like we might want to explore these parts. Where do you want to start?"

"'I must help' is really big."

"Shall we get to know it?"

"Yes."

"Great. Where is it in or around your body?"

"'I must help' is sitting on my shoulder."

"How are you feeling toward it?"

"Tender. Concerned." Jane has quickly accessed her own Self-energy.

"As the part feels your presence, see what it wants you to know."

"It is telling me, 'It is my job to look after this client. And I am failing. I can't do it.'"

"Jane, ask her, the 'I must help' part, to show you more about why she feels she must help."

Unburdening the helplessness in our last consultation meeting has eased the frozen aloneness. However, there are still parts of the six-year-old's inner world that need attention. The "I must help" part is a protector linked to the same scene. The sense of failure also needs attention. With minimal guidance from me, Jane witnesses and unburdens the six-year-old's urgent need to help and the sense that she failed to help. When this inner work is complete, the six-year-old smiles with ease and contentment; she is surrounded by light.

I invite Jane to imagine she is with her client again, and she tells me, "I feel connected to her and her pain, but not responsible. My urgency to help is gone."

Reflection

In this consultation meeting Jane completed her U-turn. She unburdened her "I must help" protector, and she witnessed and healed the feelings of helplessness and failure. Healing Jane's protectors and exiles freed Jane to give full attention to the protectors and exiles in her client. Jane's increased capacity to remain centered and calm built the foundation for a different level of work with her client. Jane expressed anticipation, even eagerness, to see her client the following week. She observed simply feeling care for her client, without any of her previous angst and frustration. She was easily able to look for an opportunity to invite her client to do her own U-turn. Jane's parts no longer distracted her. I noticed Jane's relaxed shoulders, her smile, and the strength in the vertical alignment in her body. I felt energized and excited for her.

Acknowledgment and Self-Disclosure: Owning Our Parts Out Loud

Now that the six-year-old has released her burdens, I invite Jane to consider sharing with her client the realization that, at times, her own parts interfered with her ability to remain fully present and connected. As therapists, we aspire to be fully present and accept that moments of distraction caused by our own parts are inherent in the therapeutic process. Clients generally register these breaks in connection, though not always consciously. Acknowledging even small amounts of distraction can be deeply healing for clients.

As Jane's consultant, I want to support reconnection with her client. Jane is intrigued, but this is new territory for her. She worries that mentioning her moments of distraction might not be appropriate. "So much of my training has been about *not* bringing my personal issues into the therapy relationship."

"Me too! It is important to be aware of what, how, and how much to share. However, I have come to believe that when we take responsibility for moments when our activated parts distract us or interfere in our connection with clients, we strengthen the therapeutic relationship."

I explain to Jane that owning our own parts with clients communicates a willingness to be accountable in ways that, for so many of our clients, early caretakers were not. It recognizes that even small moments of distraction can have emotional impact. A client with emotional injuries from intermittently attentive childhood caregivers often has parts that are particularly sensitive to, and vigilant about, interruptions in attention and lack of presence from people in their current life. When used sparingly and appropriately, self-disclosure models acceptance of our humanness; it becomes an invitation to self-acceptance for our clients. This kind of self-disclosure signifies a desire for the therapeutic relationship to be a collaborative one. It communicates "I am in this with you."

I ask Jane, "Does this make sense?"

Nodding, she replies, "Yes. My parts certainly were blocking me with my client!"

"And we can both guess that, even if she didn't consciously register this, she felt it. So now you have an opportunity for a 'good repair.' I have an example to illuminate my proposal. Would you like to hear it?"

"Yes."

"A dear colleague shared with me a story from her personal therapy; she gave me permission to share it. For anonymity, I have changed the names of those involved. I will refer to my colleague as Dalia, and her therapist as Eva.

"Dalia attended a workshop led by IFS founder, Richard Schwartz. While there she experienced an unburdening for one of her exiles. This had not yet occurred in her ongoing therapy. Upon return to therapy,

Dalia eagerly began to share with Eva details from the workshop and her unburdening experience. At some point during the recounting, Dalia felt that Eva was not listening; she was 'gone.'

"Dalia explained to me that she did not stop speaking, but she was worried. She noticed her thoughts: *Where did she* (Eva) *'go'? Did I do something wrong? What did I say that caused her to 'leave'?* This went on for a few minutes.

"Then Eva said, 'I want to pause for a minute. I need to let you know that for a moment or two there, when you shared your experience of unburdening, I was taken over by a part. I want to let you know that I'm back now.'

"This intervention had an immediate and profound impact on Dalia. She experienced relief; her whole body relaxed. Her internal dialogue radically shifted. She immediately felt that she was not *bad* and she had not done anything to cause Eva to 'leave.' She noticed her propensity to blame herself when there was a disconnection. With reflection, she could understand why Eva had a part step forward. Eva's openness and comfort with herself pointed to a new possibility. Eva was not lost in shame. Dalia noticed her inner critic soften; she felt more acceptance of past mistakes. Dalia recognized parts blaming herself for breaks in connection. These parts now unblended. This became a pivotal moment in her therapeutic journey.

"With this one intervention, Dalia understood that, as humans, our parts interfere in our connections. This is natural. One can accept this phenomenon without shame. We can make repair. Dalia now knew she could deeply trust that Eva was really paying attention when she was, because she was so honest when she was not. Dalia knew she could count on Eva being truthful with her. She felt her therapist's commitment to her and to their relationship. She felt treated with respect, worthy of honesty, and seen as capable of receiving it. Eva taught Dalia to notice and acknowledge parts that block connection. Dalia knew, had she been in Eva's shoes, she would have tried to hide the fact that she had 'disappeared.' She would have pretended it hadn't happened and would have quietly worked to bring herself back into connection. Dalia learned to own her parts that interfere in connection and to unblend from parts blaming and shaming her about disconnection.

"Does this make sense?"

Nodding thoughtfully, Jane answers, "This makes so much sense. I get it now."

Jane expresses interest in offering an acknowledgment to her client. We decide to role-play this intervention. I invite her to take a moment to extend Self-energy to any parts that might want to explain or defend, or any parts that might feel embarrassment or shame. Once unblended, Jane imagines she is with her client. I see and feel Jane's increased calm and confidence. I see courage. I am optimistic for both Jane and her client; I know relationships are stronger with honesty. Reconnection is possible. In our consultation time, Jane practices acknowledging her parts with her client.

Reflection

In therapy, rupture, disconnection, and mis-attunement inevitably occur. If a therapist can acknowledge such a moment without defensiveness or shame, it can become an opportunity to deepen connection and foster repair and healing (Barstow, 2005). There is an example of a simple, clear acknowledgment in the second edition of *Internal Family Systems Therapy*: "[I] just noticed one of my judgmental protectors reacting to your critic. Did you notice it, too? I've asked it to step back. I apologize" (Schwartz & Sweezy, 2020, p. 87).

Jane Integrates the Learning

In our next meeting, Jane excitedly reports the shifts she observes in herself during her session with her client. She feels connected to her client's pain and does not re-experience the intense urgency to do something or the profound helplessness. There has been some activation, but it does not blend and obscure her connection with her client. Jane acknowledged to her client that her own parts had interfered and restated her intention to be present. Her client seemed aware and accepting. Jane reported remaining calm and engaged for the entire session. She is pleased. As her consultant, I am too.

Our consultation continues. Jane observes her parts that emerge in sessions with her clients and brings them to consultation. We move comfortably between discussing client issues and further investigations of her own parts. Each time she addresses her own tangle of parts, her capacity for Self-energy expands; she returns to clinical work with an increased capacity to stay focused on her clients' needs with an open-hearted, clear attention, even when the client's distress is reminiscent of her own. Healing personal parts and professional self-disclosure positively impact therapeutic conversations. IFS calls this being, and returning to being, a Self-led therapist.

A Personal Note

As an IFS consultant, I bring my parts and my Self-energy to consultation in service of the consultee and their work with their clients. During my work with Jane, I observed and reported (as illustrated above) the subtle alterations in my physiological experience as I tracked my shifting states to confirm that my inner process supported Jane and her younger self. During the healing work with Jane's young girl, I felt warmth in my body, indicative of my Self-energy, as I appreciated the challenges the young girl experienced. As Jane was with her younger self, I extended that warmth, Self-energy, to them. Although my own history is different, I too tried to help an overwhelmed mother and failed. As Jane unburdened, a part in me recalled my own unburdening; it was as if my healed exile was encouraging Jane's six-year-old to do her healing. I knew to ask if the child carried legacy burdens in part because my young child did. My internal activation supported and informed what was needed in the consultation.

Conclusion

The role of the IFS consultant is multifaceted and moves between understanding and addressing the needs of the client and therapist and integrating the IFS processes. In this case study, the primary "presenting concern" brought to consultation ultimately became the therapist's internal activation that hindered her connection with clients. IFS consultation utilized expertise and practices often employed in IFS therapy to assist the therapist with unblending and unburdening activated parts, allowing a return to a calm, skillful, Self-led focus on the client. Additionally, the consultee was invited to consider integrating authentic self-disclosure as an important, natural process within the therapeutic relationship.

Note

1   Deep gratitude to those who supported me during the preparation of this chapter: Tema, Vicky, Emma, Lani, Patricia, Jory, Karby, Michele, Kevin, Ed, Mary, Len, Lauren, and Steve.

References

Barstow, C. (2005). *Right use of power: The heart of ethics.* Many Realms.

Schwartz, R. C. (1995). *Internal Family Systems therapy.* The Guilford Press.

Schwartz, R.C., & Sweezy, M. (2020). *Internal Family Systems therapy* (2nd ed.). The Guilford Press.

Siegel, D. J. (2007). *The mindful brain: Reflection and attunement in the cultivation of well-being.* Norton.

Sinko, A. L. (2017). Legacy Burdens. In M. Sweezy & E. L. Ziskind (Eds.), *Innovations and elaborations in Internal Family Systems therapy* (pp. 164–178). Routledge.

Van der Kolk, B. (2014). *The body keeps the score: Mind, brain and body in the transformation of trauma.* Viking Penguin.

14 In Search of Self

Emma E. Redfern

Introduction

"But what do I do about the fear?" I wondered aloud in 2012 as we were going to lunch on the last day of the group supervision module of my supervision training. I was feeling a mix of curiosity, desperation, and hope. It was as if the supervision training had enabled me more clearly to know how scared I was much of the time, how scared I was of that fear, and that I seemed somehow alone with the fear.

This chapter includes autobiographical information about how I got so scared, and how I have come to be editing and writing for a book on IFS supervision. The material that follows also touches on how hard my system has found being a supervisee. This book exists, partially, as a response to my need and desire for information and training in how to be an IFS supervisor and how to facilitate IFS supervision. The bulk of the chapter details the map or model for IFS supervision that I developed with colleague and co-author, Liz Martins, while working on this project. The chapter features disguised real-life case material used with permission.

This chapter is written by an author in the UK, where it is common practice to use the term *supervision* rather than *consultation* for what takes place between a supervisor and a supervisee, whether the latter is in training, qualified, certified, or seeking accreditation. The following terms (and their derivations) are used interchangeably: *therapy, psychotherapy,* and *counseling*. In the UK, the psychotherapy profession and its titles are not regulated by government but by various professional bodies. It has become more usual for non-psychotherapy professionals to receive supervision, and this chapter has relevance to IFS practitioners and non-psychotherapy professionals.

Adverse Childhood Experiences

Little Girl Lost: Becoming Wounded

My twin sister and I were born prematurely more than 55 years ago. This was before the term *premies* came into existence and before the practices

DOI: 10.4324/9781003044864-14

now surrounding premature birth, such as skin-to-skin kangaroo care. At birth we each needed emergency medical attention and spent our first six weeks alone in incubators. Our poor mother was unable to touch us for ten difficult days. Fast forward a few months, and mother and infants join dad on his military posting abroad, not to return "home" for two years. Really, we never returned as a family unit of four, as my father's career in the services meant he was often absent throughout my childhood. My maternal grandparents were more present in our lives, and for more than half my childhood we lived with them, or they lived with us. A family rift meant my paternal grandparents and other relatives were absent.

Such a start in life is hard for the whole family, and, although I live a life of Western, White privilege, that beginning and the adverse childhood experiences (Felitti et al., 1998) that followed (which I will not go into here) had a deep impact on me emotionally, psychologically and, especially since reaching my 50s, physiologically as I manage chronic health challenges. Looking back over my life, I see that as a child and young person I did not know who I was. I had little to no ability to access or process my emotions and bodily sensations. In many ways, I was completely alienated from and even terrified of my emotional and physical self. I frequently thought I was about to die and even tried to bring about a sort of "death through dissociation" in the hope that would make the intolerable tolerable. My system was dominated by beliefs that I was defective and that whatever was inside of me would be deadly to me (and others) if it was acknowledged and "got out." Getting sick, being in pain, having any sort of emotional response, especially fear and anger, meant I was in danger and dangerous. Such feelings had to be battled against and hidden from myself and the world. In this way I hoped I might be found acceptable and survive. Dissociating and over-containing parts worked incredibly hard. Understandably, I did not have the words to describe any of this at the time. Instead, my body often spoke for me by, for example, recurring nausea, fainting, chronic sinus problems, skin afflictions, and even one time being unable to walk with no medical explanation.

In reading Virginia M. Axline's classic psychotherapy text, *Dibs in Search of Self*, during my counseling training, I recognized aspects of my experience and process. I embarked on a search to find myself both personally and professionally. Since embracing IFS, this has expanded into a search for Self, and each of these meanings are alluded to in the title of this chapter.

Becoming a Client and Integrative Therapist

In May of the year I turned 31, life as I knew it metaphorically blew apart. Up until then, my valiant protectors had enabled me to function as an apparently normal and successful person. However, on that fateful day in May, my system was rendered a blow that made ineffective the ways of coping of parts I now know of as protectors. An outside-in fire burnt my flat down, and I and the occupants of the nine flats were homeless for ten months. I was literally rescued by a fireman and his ladder from the hideous fiery death that exiles had already been reliving over and over in their imaginations since I was six years old. At six, I had visited my father in hospital, where a nearby patient suffered from having been thrown on a bonfire. Now, as an adult, my protectors could no longer keep the exiles from storming the gates. I dissolved into hysterical tears at the sounds of a fire engine or its siren, my ability to eat and hydrate faltered, parts feared suicidal parts would use the ultimate solution to make it all stop. I could no longer keep what was on the inside locked away and out of sight, and I felt helpless to intrusion and invasion by things on the outside. Thankfully, three years later a trauma-informed solicitor spotted signs of PTSD (post-traumatic stress disorder) and secured an insurance settlement, which enabled me to attend a group psychotherapy program for those diagnosed with PTSD. From that first experience of therapy, I was hooked and have been a client "on and off" ever since, making positive use of various forms of therapy and many therapeutic relationships.

Reclaiming Myself: Feeling Safe Enough in Therapy

Without the fire, I might not have been "ripe for therapy" and might not have fallen in love with accompanied inner work in such a wholehearted way. Another therapeutic relationship I have been blessed to discover since the fire was that with my husband. On marrying, we moved to the Southwest of England and started a new life together, which included me enrolling in a Humanistic Integrative counseling training. The desire to be a professional therapist was multifarious: to counter or balance the tendency of my parts toward avoidance, to give to others what I had not received, and to legitimize my continued search in therapy for earned secure attachment and ways to be more than the fear and shame I was filled with.

The presence of trauma in my system has propelled me on a particular personal therapy journey and along a specific trajectory of training in protocol-driven trauma therapies. This has partly been due to a growing awareness that much "talking therapy" fails to address trauma, so that if exiles unburden, it is almost by accident rather than by design. Using EMDR (eye movement desensitization and reprocessing) and, more recently, IFS, I have found ways to explicitly and safely work with trauma, consistently move beyond the fear of the fear, and access Self's ability to unburden exiles in my own and my clients' systems.

Wounded Healers

You may be wondering why I am focusing on client experience in a chapter on supervision. This is partly because I am not alone in being a wounded-healer therapist (St. Arnaud, 1997; Wheeler 2007). According to the Traumatic Stress Research Consortium (TSRC) at the Kinsey Institute Indiana University, the preliminary results from a survey of trauma clinicians "lend support to a narrative in which the majority of trauma professionals are also trauma survivors" (Kinsey Institute Traumatic Stress Research Consortium, 2020, p. 8). The frequency and number of reported adverse childhood experiences (ACEs) was higher than in the overall US population, with 86.63 percent of trauma professionals reporting at least one ACE, compared to 67 percent in the overall population. The figure for trauma professionals reporting three or more ACEs was 58.14 percent compared to 22 percent in the overall population. Childhood maltreatment was measured by self-report using the Childhood Trauma Questionnaire and revealed that trauma workers had higher rates of (or at least conscious awareness of) emotional abuse, sexual abuse, and emotional neglect histories when compared with data from a general sample in the US.

Losing Myself: Feeling Unsafe in Supervision

Understandably, with a history like mine, I learned to fear more than trust people and was often blended with dedicated protectors as a supervisee in supervision. I developed many shame protectors. Most notably, Drama Triangle (Karpman, 1968; Hughes & Pengelly, 1997), overly compliant (Rennie, 1994), dissociative, and co-narcissistic (Rappoport, 2005) parts. Such parts actively prevented other parts of me from speaking up (internally and externally) and showing up in the supervisory relationship when the relationship seemed unsafe. These shame protectors also struggled around giving feedback to supervisors, such that my needs might be met. To suggest that someone else might be getting things wrong for me sometimes still evokes shame in my system, which distorts or reverses the inadequacy so that I am the one who feels at fault.

Feeling anxious or unsafe in supervision is not a new concept, and many authors have written about how supervisees (Gilbert & Evans, 2000) and supervisors (Hawthorne, 1975) may consciously or unconsciously manage their anxiety in supervision. This is done by what Kadushin & Harkness (2014) call playing games, and what IFS might call leading with protectors.

Thankfully, my professional body embraces a culture of supervision and expects me to have monthly supervision for the duration of my active career. This has given me the time and space to work at showing up in supervision. Training as a supervisor myself has helped my system seek and find support and resourcing as supervisee and supervisor, and I am now more able to experience supervision as enjoyable and impactful.

Becoming a Parts-Aware Supervisor

Learning about Transactional Analysis (TA) and Karpman's Drama Triangle (Karpman, 1968) during my psychotherapy training, together with Voice

Dialogue therapy, introduced me to the concept of human multiplicity. Over 20 years later, I still find it helpful to recognize the activity of protectors characterized by the three roles of Victim, Rescuer, and Persecutor (see Figure 14.1). Generally, the Drama Triangle is written about and conceived of as an interpersonal dynamic (Hughes & Pengelly, 1997). However, I also conceive of these dynamics as happening intrapersonally in different ways, an example of which can be seen in Schwartz's account of client Quinn (Schwartz & Sweezy, 2020, pp. 11–12).

In IFS terms, a crucial function of these rescuer-victim-persecutor dynamics is to keep attention away from personal vulnerability or exiles and the taking of personal responsibility. Instead, the focus is on the other actors (internal and external) on the drama triangle(s). This "other" focus is one of the reasons I like to share with clients and teach supervisees the Healthy Triangle alongside the Drama Triangle (see Redfern, 2021), because it brings the focus back onto the person themselves and who and how they are. Adapted from the Beneficial Triangle (Proctor & Tehrani, 2001), the Healthy Triangle (see Figure 14.2) references ways of being or qualities of a person who has access to Self: vulnerable, potent (in the sense of having personal power, choice, and agency), and responsive to and responsible for oneself. *Vulnerable* in the Brené Brown (2017) sense of a healthily vulnerable person having the courage to be aware of their own wounding, while remaining open-hearted and accepting of their own needs and emotions *and* those of others. The Healthy Triangle provides a mini map of where successful therapy might be headed as well as details how a supervisee and supervisor might be characterized when accessing Self-energy.

Professionals having a common understanding of the Drama Triangle can be helpful in recognizing hidden dynamics, and sharing the Healthy Triangle can be helpful in exploring what mental health might look like (Redfern, 2021). However, there is no road map within Integrative psychotherapy for how to move from one triangle to the other, and it is left up to the individual practi-

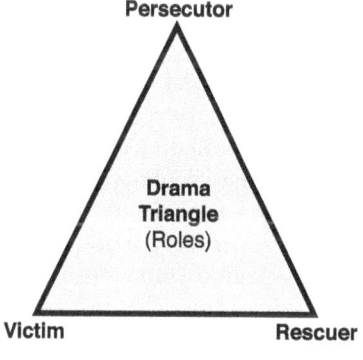

Figure 14.1 The Drama Triangle

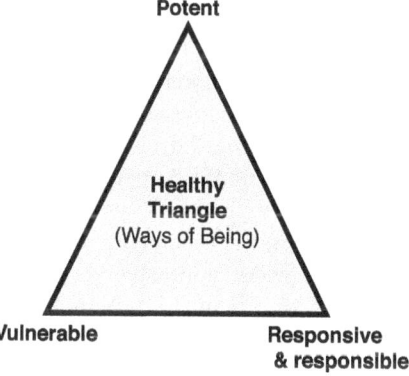

Figure 14.2 The Healthy Triangle

tioner and person to determine how movement happens. Alternatively, practitioners can trust that this growth will happen automatically and gradually as part of a successful therapeutic process. Fortunately, professionals and individuals now have IFS ways of engaging with extreme protectors, such as rescuers, persecutors, and victims, with the potential to discover and address their fears, heal the wounds of those they protect, and unburden parts who are burdened.

Becoming an IFS Supervisor

Having fallen in love with the IFS model from first reading "the red book," as the first edition of *Internal Family Systems Therapy* is known (Schwartz, 1995), I enjoy practicing IFS, especially getting to know protectors' positive intentions for their system and asking what they are afraid might happen if they didn't do their (often) life-or-death jobs. IFS puts front and centre the fear at the heart of the human condition in a way that is normalizing, helpful, and transformative. Thanks to experiencing the Self of the IFS model, I know from the inside that Self doesn't "do fear" and can be with fearful parts. Organically, I began bringing IFS into my supervision relationships and practice. This has been challenging to my system, not least because I have parts who prefer to read the book and do the training before doing anything "for real," and there was no IFS supervision book and there was no training. Also, my experience of receiving IFS consultation from a US consultant, as transformative as it was, also brought confusion, as it seemed indistinguishable from IFS therapy. I had no road map for how that might be possible, acceptable, or even if it was desirable for me to offer that as a UK supervisor.

Introducing a Model of IFS Supervision: The 8 Facets

Having trained independently with the Centre for Supervision and Team Development, Bath and London, Liz Martins and I have both been developing our own maps or models to guide, hold, and help us reflect on and explain our supervision work to ourselves and to others. In Chapter 3, Liz Martins introduces "The Fs and Ps of IFS Supervision," and in the remainder of this chapter, I briefly introduce a map or model that we hope functions for IFS supervision similarly to how the seven-eyed model of Hawkins and Shohet (2012) functions for the helping professions.

The 8 Facets of IFS Supervision are: (1) Self, (2) the client's system, (3) the therapist's/supervisee's system, (4) the supervisor's system, (5) the IFS model itself, (6) the therapeutic relationship; (7) the supervisory relationship; and (8) the wider context(s). For a visual representation summarizing all eight facets, see Figure 14.3. Note that this is not a linear model – each facet influences and is connected to all the others; the map is not the territory; every supervision session may not feature each facet; it is worth considering if there is one facet that dominates or if any are neglected; and different facets may be more applicable than others for therapists and practitioners at the beginning of their journey with IFS, compared to more seasoned IFS professionals. This material arises out of supervision of therapeutic work with individual adults. However, the model can be adapted for use in group supervision; in supervision of those who work with children, young people, and couples; and in non-clinical settings. To relate the following material to practice, I may refer to material in previous chapters, cite clinical examples from my own practice, and, for each facet, I include possible supervision questions that supervisors and supervisees might ask inside themselves and of each other.

Inspired by Schwartz's vision of humanity and our interconnectedness, I hope that this model, this chapter, and this book will contribute an understanding that how we gaze and where we look from are important, as is what we see and choose to focus upon. As a prelude to introducing the first facet, I remind us:

> When we're in Self, we remember our connectedness to our parts, to other people, and to the Earth. We view each other as sacred beings and relate with love and respect. We also remember our connectedness to the SELF and can receive wise guidance from that level of consciousness. In being Self-led, we find our vision naturally and act on it … And we increase the field of Self on the planet and work to reduce the fields of burdens that engulf it.
>
> (Schwartz, 2021, p. 189)[1]

Facet 1: Self

Unsurprisingly, when I introduce the 8 Facets, I begin with Self. Being able to access this way of "being with" is the game changer at the heart of the IFS model. Self is depicted in Figure 14.3 as a large outer circle, representing the container and containment of Larger Self, and a smaller circle, similarly shaded, within each IFS triangle (Sykes, 2017), representing each of the three participants of supervision (Hughes & Pengelly, 1997).

An overarching goal of IFS Supervision, as with IFS therapy, is an increase in Self-leadership for all three participants of supervision (client, therapist, supervisor). IFS Supervision can have many similarities to IFS therapy as it seeks to support greater access to Self within the supervisee's system using in-sight, direct access, and the usual means of unblending (as shown throughout the book and in Dan Reed and Ray Wooten's Appendix).

However, Self does not exist within a vacuum, nor does access to it turn us all into clones of each other, as highlighted by the diversity and rich individual offerings from each of the authors and author pairings in this book. As Tamala Floyd (Chapter 6), Mary Steege (Chapter 10), and Sharon Cooper and Kimberly Corey (Chapter 11), especially, make clear, certain professions, milieu, and experiences of suffering affect how our parts develop, configure, and

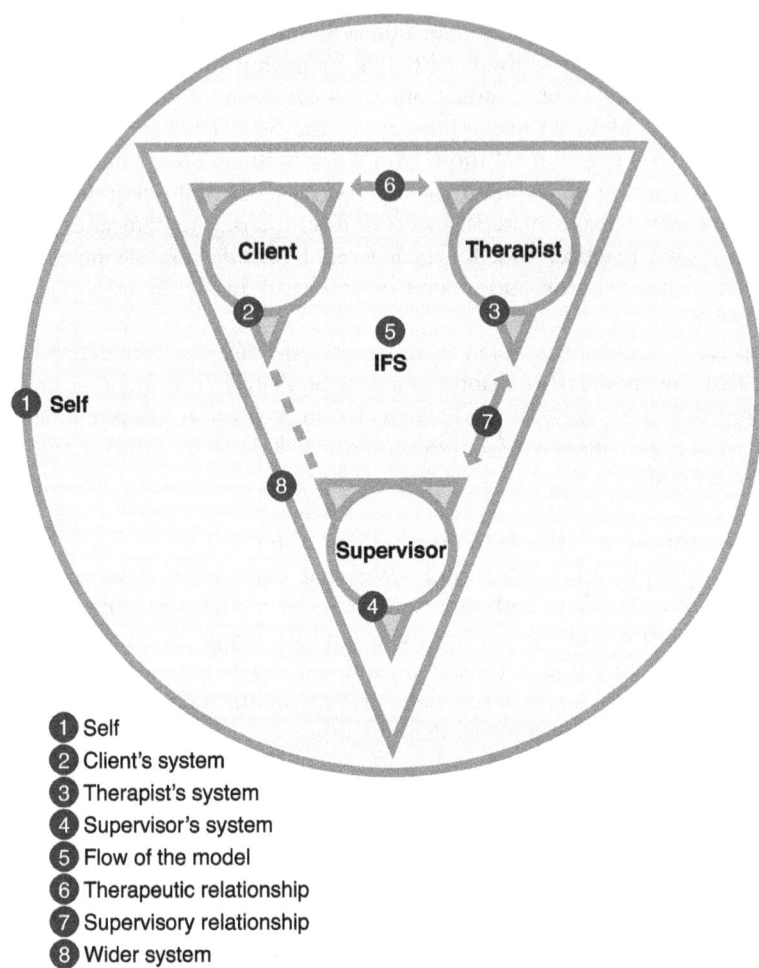

Figure 14.3 The 8 Facets of IFS Supervision
Source: © 2020 Liz Martins and Emma E. Redfern. Used by permission.

present in therapy. Similarly, access to Self does not make a person infallible and beyond reproach. Self-leadership, as Fran Booth (Chapter 13) points out, is a process, it fluctuates and, when connection to one's Self is lost, it affects connection to the other, and relational repair may be needed.

The nature of Facet 1 supervision varies depending on the experience and stage of development of the supervisee, the stage of development of the supervisory relationship, and the task in hand. The main purpose of this facet is to keep as central to IFS therapy the healing and transformative presence of Self (which makes the practice of IFS stand out from "working with parts" featured in other non–IFS models and practices).

Facet 1 supervision questions include:

- How does Self show up in my life, my supervisees' lives, their clients' lives?
- Do parts allow Self to speak for them?
- Does the client have access to Self in sessions, or are you mostly using implicit and explicit direct access?
- Now you have presented the work with your client, shall we enquire who needs or wants attention inside you from the "you who is not a part"?

Facet 2: The Client's System

Using this lens or focus, the supervisee and I attend to the client's system of parts (managers, firefighters, and exiles) and access to Self (see Figure 14.4) as noticed and, usually, presented by the supervisee. We take note of who in the internal system might have brought the client to therapy and what triggered this. We notice any polarized parts who might not want to be in therapy, and who in the wider systems might feel threatened that the client is in therapy. We bear in mind that some parts, especially exiles, may not know the client is in therapy, and many parts will not know Self well or not know of Self's existence. We notice exile and protector beliefs and hold curiosity as to how they may impact on the therapy.

We also attend to the client's wider context and the impact of and relationships with parts in siblings, parents, partners, dependants, colleagues, bosses, carers, etc. (without being seduced into treating people who are not in the therapy room). Looking out for and enquiring about the presence of legacy burdens, unattached burdens, and cultural burdens may feature here.

Facet 2 supervision questions include:

- Who in the client brought them to therapy? Are parts in other people's systems invested in the client seeking therapy?
- Who in the client's system might you not be aware of?
- How much Self is available within the client's system?
- What burdened beliefs are showing up in the client's system, and how might these impact on the process of therapy?

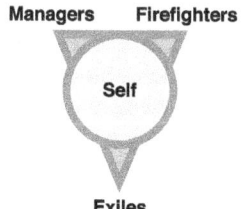

Figure 14.4 The IFS Triangle
Source: Adapted from Cece Sykes, LCSW, 2017, p. 30. Used by permission.

The main purpose of this aspect of supervision is to help the supervisee, where needed, to flesh out the client's system of parts and Self, paying particular attention to any therapist blind spots, biases, and assumptions.

After introducing the next facet, I share case material of "a match" in client and therapist of what I think of as Drama Triangle parts.

Facet 3: The Therapist's (Supervisee's) System

The main purposes of this aspect of supervision are:

- To help the supervisee relate to their parts so the supervisee can engage with clients with more Self-energy available.
- To assist the supervisee in using awareness of their own parts' activation as a source of potential information about the client.

The system of the therapist is represented with the same triangle (Sykes, 2017) and circle as the client's system (Figure 14.4) but appears to the right in the larger diagram (Figure 14.3). Using this lens or focus, I attend to the supervisee's system of parts as they show up or are triggered in the work with clients and as they show up or are triggered in supervision. I help supervisees track and attend to their own parts and speak for them as necessary in the therapeutic and supervisory relationships (see Chapter 13 for how to acknowledge and speak for parts who have contributed to a break in connection with the other). We also attend to the supervisee's wider context and the impact on their internal system from outside by, for example, managers within their training establishment or employment.

For supervisees transitioning from an existing modality to IFS or integrating IFS into an existing way of working, attention may need to be given to therapist parts invested in old ways of working or who have yet to meet, trust, and, if applicable, negotiate a working alliance with Self.

We attend to the supervisee's access to Self and how this varies with different clients as well as to points in supervision where parts may become active. We use IFS approaches to aid the therapist in unblending and may go on to work therapeutically with therapist parts, if contracted for and done in the service of the client. Personally, I take care not to unconsciously shift the supervisory relationship to a primarily therapeutic relationship. In my view, such a shift is not advisable. It runs the risk of perpetuating a one-up:one-down relationship in which the supervisee may feel pressure to continually produce a wound to work on (thus exacerbating the risk of drama triangle rescuer-victim dynamics). Ideally, supervision provides space for professional competence and capability to grow. When working with beginners, particularly, I enjoy making room for supervisees to bring their confusion, share curiosity about the model, practice aspects of IFS together (such as direct access), and explore how to transition from previous ways of working to using IFS. Also, at a practical level of resources here in the UK, access to reasonably-priced IFS therapy is potentially greater than access to reasonably-priced IFS supervision. I like to think supervisees get something different and more than IFS therapy in our work together. Other supervisors and consultants will have different preferences, and offerings in this area and supervisees can, hopefully, have some choice about who they wish to work with, in which ways, and to what depth (see Chapter 2 by Reed and Wooten).

Facet 3 questions for supervisor and supervisee include:

- How does the therapist feel toward the client?
- Which therapist parts are blocking or impacting on the work with this client?
- What supervisee parts show up regularly in supervision?
- What are parts too frightened of saying to the supervisor (or to the supervisee)?
- Who might I not be seeing or hearing from in the supervisee?

Meeting a Supervisee's Drama Triangle Protectors

Eliza is an Integrative psychotherapist who, at the time of writing, is attending an online IFS Institute Level 1 training. Eliza is also a wounded healer with what I think of as Drama Triangle protectors, and we have a shared understanding of the Drama and Healthy Triangles. She and the client (respectively) seem, in my view, to alternate between two dances Rescuer-Victim and Victim-Persecutor. In my opinion, rescuer-persecutor-victim dynamics were set up from the beginning when the client stated, "I won't do any of that shutting my eyes, going inside," and a part or parts in the supervisee (for whatever good reasons of their own) agreed to that without exploration and curiosity.

At first, the supervisee was able to access her own Self-energy when with the client. Recently, frustrated parts have begun to blend, and they suggest to Eliza that she ends the relationship with the client. This is partly because the client says therapy is not working, she does not feel any better, and partly because, as Eliza puts it, "She won't do IFS." I address the latter point first, not to correct the supervisee, but as a form of hope merchanting, suggesting that therapy may not be going as badly as it seems.

"Okay, Eliza, I understand how frustrated you feel at the client 'not doing' IFS. However, the way I look at it, she is doing IFS in that she is speaking from and showing you parts of her who are in conflict. From what you've told me about her, these include:

(a) A part who is frightened of going inside and told you she won't do so.
(b) A part asking for your help/rescue when she relates her latest upset.

(c)　A controlling part who dominates much of the time.

(d)　A 'do nothing' part who says being controlling is wrong.

(e)　A part she reports as 'having a meltdown.'

To me, it sounds like these might be Drama Triangle protectors who are trying to manage and avoid her distress at all costs. Does that fit at all?"

"It does yes."

"And it seems to me that parts of you are 'joining her on the Drama Triangle,' which is to join with her avoidance of her wounds – her exiles – and her vulnerability." (The supervisee nods and seems relieved.) "I am wondering who is currently driving your inner psychic bus when you are with this client. Would you be willing to go inside and find out?"

(Eliza is willing to go inside and finds a relevant protector.)

"I see a 16-year-old girl who looks like me."

"How do you feel toward her, Eliza?"

"I'm curious and want to know what's up."

"Okay, great, ask her what she fears about this client."

"I hear, *Don't push the client, she'll unravel and that's really scary.*"

(The unwillingness of this part to tolerate distress or vulnerability signals to me that this part has qualities of a Rescuer.)

"Does that make sense to you?"

"Yes, this part says her job is to care for older people, especially women, and be nice and kind to them."

"Okay, anything else she would like you to know about this?"

"She says she's frightened I'll get angry with the client, or the client will get angry with me."

(Parts who have rescuing qualities often fear angry parts inside and out and work hard to pacify or block them.)

"Does that make some sense as well?"

"Yes. This part was a rebellious teenager and feels guilty about all that she put her mother through. ... That's it."

"Okay, great."

(It seems this part has changed from being more persecutory in the past. It is also possible the active part is referring to another part. The details are not important now, and instead of continuing with the witnessing, which seems complete anyway, I ask Eliza to update this part about Eliza's job.)

"I wonder, does this part know you are a therapist now, and that your job is to help people go to their pain safely and be with it?"

"... No, she didn't know that."

"Fair enough. So go ahead and update her some more and see how she responds."

"... I hear, *You're brave* and *You can do that without me, I don't want to be involved.*"

"Let her know you get that."

(After a moment or two …) "Does that work for you that she isn't there when you work with this client?"

"Yes, sure, that feels much better when I think of working with this client next time."

Thankfully, my own Drama Triangle parts were not triggered, and thanks to IFS we were able to facilitate the supervisee going inside to alleviate some of the strain in her system, which was mirroring the strain and conflict in the client's system. It would have been all too easy for me to blend with a Rescuer part, *I'll tell Eliza what to do to make it better*, or a Persecutor part, who might have let her frustration show: *She keeps bringing this client to supervision!* Alternatively, this could have triggered painful exile beliefs in me (and potentially the supervisee), *Something's not working right, it's my fault, and I don't know how to fix it*. This brings us to the next facet – the supervisor's system.

Facet 4: The Supervisor's System

Here the attention is on the supervisor's here-and-now experience in supervision: what parts are activated in relation to the supervisee, in response to the material being shared, and in response to the client as experienced by the supervisor. This system is represented by the same IFS triangle (Sykes, 2017) as for the client and therapist (see Figure 14.4). In the diagram of the 8 Facets (Figure 14.3), Facet 4 is represented by the bottom triangle, together with a dotted line joining the supervisor's system and the client's system. Although supervisor and client only rarely meet directly in the external world, internally and energetically I still create connection to supervisee's clients and remain open to information inside my system about that. I then consider if and how to use any information that arises for me, whether to keep it to myself or offer to share it with the supervisee. For an interesting example of choosing what to share, see Pamela Krause and the case example of Philip (Chapter 4). There, as the therapist presents the case, Krause shares with the reader, and not with the therapist, her parts' responses, while she does share with the therapist her own parts' responses from putting herself in the shoes of the client's mother.

When supervising, I have choices about how to respond to my parts' activation. I may seek to unblend in the session and have my activated parts give space. Where helpful, I may choose to speak for my own vulnerable or protector parts. This helps normalize multiplicity, model transparency, and allows me also to be human. Often, risking speaking for one of my parts may enable a supervisee to recognize in themselves a similar or opposing reaction and loosen any tension around having such a part. Ann Drouilhet (Chapter 5) shares an example of this happening in her consultation with Sivan.

Where I identify trailheads for myself, I may work with those trailheads later, alone or with peers, or with a supervisor of supervision to enable more

Self-presence. In addition, I will be seeking to determine if/how parts' activation is communicating important information about the client, the supervisee, or the therapeutic and supervisory relationships. Nancy Wonder (Chapter 8) writes about this in terms of making the unconscious conscious. Hawkins and Shohet (2012, p. 102) write as follows:

> I must know when I am normally tired, bored, fidgety, fearful, sexually aroused, tensing my stomach, etc., in order to ascertain that this eruption is not entirely my own inner process bubbling away, but is a received import. In this process, the unconscious material of the supervisee is being received by the unconscious receptor of the supervisor, and the supervisor is tentatively bringing this material into consciousness for the supervisee to explore.

As an IFS supervisor, I may choose to lean into certain activities which, depending on their origin and execution, may be Self-led, parts-led, or arise from a partnership between Self and part or parts:

- Teaching by sharing experience and knowledge, and modeling how to do IFS;
- Creatively using role-play, psychodrama, externalizing, and other techniques;
- Encouraging, including validating the therapist's system and their work with clients;
- Evaluating competence collaboratively with the supervisee; or
- Supportively inquiring about the supervisee's self-care and well-being.

The main purposes of this aspect of supervision are to assist the supervisor:

- In maintaining access to Self; and
- In accessing and making use of information from their own parts' activation, which may provide a source of potential information not only about the supervisee and the client, but also about any stakeholders, real and potential.

Facet 4 supervision questions supervisors could ask themselves include:

- Is my configuration of Self and parts a good fit for this supervisee and their system (as far as I am aware) for the supervision task in hand and in our supervision relationship?
- What parts are showing up in my system right now?
- Are the parts activated in me providing information about the here and now, the therapeutic dyad, and/or trailheads connected to my own history?

- What parts do I hide in supervision, and on what parts do I rely?
- What do parts of me least want this supervisee to think, believe, or say about me?
- How do I feel toward the supervisee/their client?

Supervisor U-Turn Required

Thanks to many years of therapy, my system is becoming less dominated by Drama Triangle protectors. However, I can still be more parts-led in supervision than I would like. My parts have often become activated when they perceive that parts in supervisees have come to supervision to get answers from me about the client's system. I realize that Schwartz's text about clients being tor-mentors to therapists also fits supervisees and supervisors:

> Between sessions, I will follow up by bringing the parts who my [supervisee] aroused to my own [supervision/self-reflection] to give them attention. In this way our [supervisees] become our *tor-mentors*— by tormenting us, they mentor us, making us aware of who in us needs our loving attention.
>
> (Schwartz, 2013, p. 17; my adaptations in square brackets)

In the following example, I am providing IFS supervision to a therapist trained in Integrative psychotherapy with a leaning toward the psychodynamic. She has completed online IFS training, and I am her first IFS supervisor. Initially, I believe, like many of us, she struggled with what I think of as the professional deconstruction and reconstruction necessary to shift from one way of working to another. I empathize with the struggle, reminding myself of the benefit I have received in previously going through a professional deconstruction and reconstruction process when I trained in protocol-based, client-led EMDR before subsequently training in IFS.

Judgmental parts of me are becoming activated, and because it is early in our relationship, I choose not to speak for them, fearing a rupture of the relationship. This is also because my Self has not yet met these parts, and I am unsure I could speak to her for them not from them. In between appointments, I decide to do some self-supervision, adapting for intrapsychic use a three-step assertion message formulation that is usually used interpersonally (Bolton, 1979). The original formulation is a way to communicate the impact on the speaker of a specific behaviour by the other that the speaker would like changed. However, the speaker does not take responsibility for if and how the change occurs. The message is structured in three steps, which involve completing three sentence stems:

- Step one communicates the perceived boundary-breaking behaviour: "When you …"

- Step two communicates the emotional response(s) of the speaker: "I feel ..."
- Step three communicates the real-world impact of the behaviour (such as being late for work): "Because ..."

I choose to go inside to hear from parts reacting to a statement the supervisee uses frequently, which is shown in the center of Figure 14.5. Instead of imagining speaking to the supervisee, I have the parts communicate with me by completing the sentence stems: "When she ... I feel ... Because. ..."

Later, a similar issue arises in another supervisory relationship with an Integratively-trained supervisee "with a part who is person-centered." He

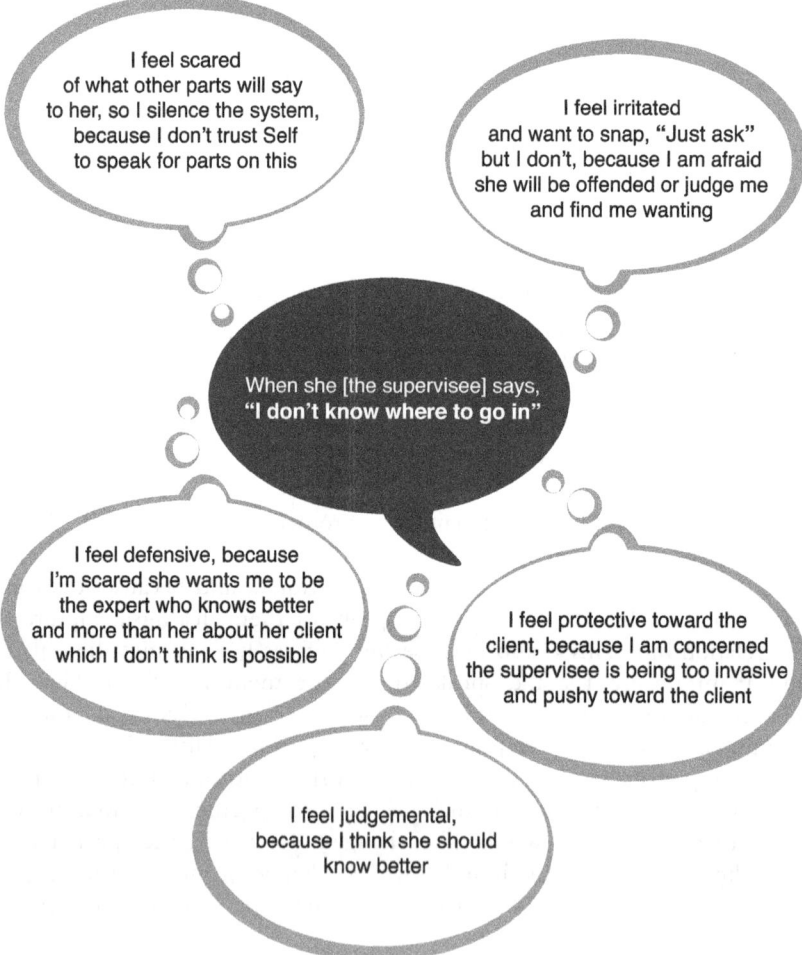

Figure 14.5 Supervisor's Parts Map

has attended a day's Introduction to IFS and completed some IFS reading. This time, having already listened to my parts, I feel less reactive, and I respond in a more Self-led way, validating the part of the supervisee who doesn't know where to begin using IFS with one of his clients.

"I don't know which part to start with."

"That makes sense to me. Why would you know which part to start with? If this were regular talking therapy, would you believe you should know which part to start with?"

"No."

"And it's no different now. Possibly because IFS uses protocols and has a structure and a flow, it might seem like you should know which part to start with? And you may have ideas and could offer those, but ..."

(The supervisee interrupts with an Aha! moment) "The client can still be the expert on their process and experience, like in Rogerian therapy."

"Absolutely. Perhaps the part who doesn't know could relax and let you be curious with your client about who needs attention first?"

"Yes, and there's some relief around that inside."

Facet 5: The IFS Healing Journey/Flow of the Model

Facet 5 is represented in the center of Figure 14.3 by the letters "IFS." Where the therapist is working to the IFS model, the focus here is on the therapist's technical understanding of and ability to use the IFS model with clients and with their own system. In my experience, this is one of the lenses through which supervisor and supervisee most frequently gaze when the supervisee is in training or recently graduated from Level 1. The main purpose of this aspect of supervision is to increase the therapist's ability in mastering and delivering the protocols of IFS, such as explicit direct access, helping clients go inside, hope merchanting, and so on. As is made clear throughout the rest of the book, to achieve these things, the supervisee may need to prioritize attending to parts in themselves who are getting in the way of the work of learning and implementing IFS. Supervision is one of the places and relationships in which this can happen.

Where the supervisee is not familiar with the IFS model, the supervisor may need to use different language and concepts more familiar to the therapist. However, the IFS model may still provide a guide to the non-IFS therapy process by, for example, getting to know and appreciating protectors and gaining their permission before approaching wounded parts (Liz Martins refers to this in Chapter 3).

Facet 5 supervision questions include:

- (When the supervisee is not IFS trained) Which aspects of IFS are relevant in the supervisory relationship and in the therapeutic work?
- Where in the flow of the model does the IFS therapist or practitioner feel confident and clear?

- Where in the steps of healing is there confusion or challenge?
- How is stuckness to be worked with and attended to?

Reed and Wooten (Chapter 2), Martins (Chapter 3), and the interview with Schwartz (Chapter 1) have much to say on working with stuckness. In my experience, a number of areas impede the flow of the model and/or contribute to some therapists' and some practitioners' stuckness some of the time, including:

- Poor or no contracting, and contracting that does not take multiplicity into account;
- Therapists not doing deep personal work to access Self and experience the model from the inside;
- Inability or unwillingness of therapists to reflect on their competencies; or
- Parts of the therapist or practitioner remaining committed to previous ways of working rather than taking a risk on trusting Self and practicing IFS.

The main purpose of this aspect of supervision is to focus on the learning and application of IFS by the therapist/practitioner/other professional and, to an extent, the client. This may include the supervisor teaching, modeling, and facilitating aspects of IFS. This facet attends to accessing Self-energy within the IFS framework.

Facet 6: The Therapeutic Relationship

In Figure 14.3, Facet 6 is represented at the top of the diagram by the horizontal line joining the client's system and the therapist's system. This facet calls on the therapist to assess the "pH" of the therapeutic dyad. The human body maintains a healthy balance of acidity and alkalinity, which is measured by pH level. I use the idea of a pH level and note that IFS supervisors, therapists, and practitioners strive to keep balanced attention both inside their own systems and on the external system(s). This balance of dual attention is represented in Figure 14.6, which shows the capital letter H or "psychotherapeutic H," with the vertical sidebars representing the internal, vertical Self-to-part and part-to-Self relating inside each person. The horizontal crossbar represents the various permutations of the Self-to-Self, part-to-Self, and part-to-part connections moving between the client and therapist.

Facet 6 supervision questions include:

- Can the client achieve Self-to-part relationship within their own system during therapy sessions?
- Can the supervisee relate to the client from Self and have their own activated parts relax when requested?

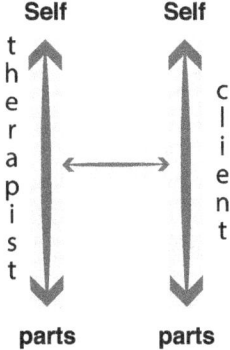

Figure 14.6 The Therapeutic Dyad and the Psychotherapeutic H (pH)

- If you imagine asking your client who you are to them, what do you imagine the client might say?

What follows is an excerpt from a supervision session featuring a therapeutic relationship in which the pH of the therapeutic relationship could be described as out of balance and needing attention. Supervision includes attending to the vertical or Self-to-part relationship inside the supervisee, with a view to aiding the supervisee to be their own "I" in the storm – and the client also.

An Alliance of Client and Therapist Protectors

A supervision session with Ivana, a Level 3 trained IFS practitioner, provides an example of attending to Facet 6, the therapeutic relationship. Note that this is not necessarily how I would work in a new supervisory relationship when we were just getting to know each other. Ivana and I have built up a trusting and enjoyable supervisory relationship online over six months, and her skills in case conceptualization and contracting are progressing. In this example, she brings to supervision her sense of being stuck in the work with Paddy, a successful amateur sportsman and part-time model. Ivana tells me the client has a harsh and obsessive inner critic worried about the client's age and potentially declining looks and sports prowess. It makes him work out all the time and wear the latest trends and use top products. This part holds strong beliefs about what men should look like and seems polarized with another part who keeps checking in the mirror and fearfully wondering, *Do I look grotesque? Have I always been such a monster?* These parts have a lot of power, and at times Ivana agrees to turn her chair away and not look directly at Paddy. Wanting to get some sense of whether the supervisee has used this and other content to conceptualize the case in terms of protectors and exiles, I ask Ivana, "Who do you think, or who has told you they brought Paddy to therapy?"

"Well, his father is a psychotherapist, and he's always been into psychology, and he's got this analytical part who works really hard in therapy."

"Tell me more, can you?"

"This part knows all the parts and their beliefs and relationships, and we map them together."

(Getting the sense that protectors are dominating the work, I enquire to see if Self in the client is in relation to protectors as they share or if something else is happening.) "How do you get this information? Is it through in-sight or direct access?"

"Neither. The client can't do in-sight, and I don't like doing direct access. It's a part that informs about the system intellectually. It also tells the client's story – of how his younger brother was disfigured in an accident, and how he thinks his parents pitied the brother behind his back thinking he was ugly. The client didn't want to be thought ugly too, so he got into keeping in shape as a sportsman and then the modeling during his gap year before Uni, and beautiful women have always been attracted to him and …"

"Okay, great. And what's 'the beautifier' afraid would happen if it didn't keep him in shape and attractive?"

"It's afraid he'll become suicidal or reclusive when he gets rejected and attacked."

"And does it make sense to you and him that parts fear being rejected and attacked?"

"I don't know. He doesn't know."

(Sensing that the supervisee has amassed a lot of helpful information that she doesn't know what to do with, I am drawn to pursuing awareness of the nature of parts.) "Okay. From your understanding of how IFS works and the categories of parts, what's your guess?"

"The feeling grotesque …?"

"Yes?" (After a pause, and waiting for more that doesn't come, I continue) "As you were talking, I kept being reminded of 'Beauty and the Beast,' and how the beast isn't what he seems. The client's sense of being a monster seems key. My guess is there is a wounded exile that the system fears is a monster and is determined to keep away out of sight. If so, that exile is in need of a relationship to Self and of healing."

"It's helpful to hear you say it so clearly. It's like I knew it, but it was a long way away in a foggy place, locked away and unusable."

"Interesting. We'll come to that. Meanwhile, can I share the other image I've been getting?"

(I have a very visual mind, and I often have an awareness of what is "in the field" from images that arise. If an image persistently shows itself, I am likely to share it (Shohet & Shohet, 2021).)

"Yes, please."

"In my mind's eye, I see Self at the top in a circle, like the sun, then there is a barrier between Self and the exiles, which keeps Self away from them." (The supervisee gives a sigh of relief and nods when I pause to see that it is okay for me to carry on.) "I'm picking up that the work you are doing with the client's 'part-that-knows-all-about-the-system' is building a brick wall keeping the client's Self and your Self away from any vulnerability. And we both know this is the job of protectors. It's like each part you discuss is another brick in that wall. You are both expertly gaining lots of information at the protector level, which isn't leading to healing, inner relationships with and connection to Self." (The supervisee seems moved.) "How is that for you to hear?"

"A relief. Yes, that feels absolutely right. Where do I start to do it differently?"

"If it was me, I would want to see if the client's 'part-that-knows-all-about-the-system' is willing to meet and trust the client's Self and cede control and grant permission for Self to go to any wounded ones it protects."

"I'm just recalling the client did access some vulnerability at one point. He cried once in session and said it felt really positive to be able to do that."

"That's a great recollection. So, the client may be up for accessing some vulnerability and exile energy?" (Supervisee nods.) "How would it be if we turned to your system now? My sense is you knew all of what those images conveyed to us both."

"Yes, I did, but I couldn't make use of the awareness."

"Alright, who keeps this out of reach? Who keeps it foggy in there, or …?" (The supervisee closes her eyes and turns inward with curiosity.)

"Ah, it's my intellectual, hardworking therapist part."

"Yes? Do you see the part in there? (She nods) Ask the part what it's afraid would happen if it didn't work so hard."

"I'm very blended with it. Can you do direct access?"

"Sure." (Agreeing to explicit direct access, I welcome the part.) "Welcome."

(The supervisee's part is eager to speak and be heard.)

"I dread what I'm going to see and hear, and I don't want to fail the client. The client's part really wants to understand the system and gather all that information, and I'm happy to help it do that." (The supervisee's therapist part has formed an alliance with the client's 'part-that-knows-all-about-the-system.')

"Well, that makes a lot of sense to me, and I feel moved and appreciative that you are willing to speak to me about this."

"And I don't know how to get those other parts in the client to trust me or trust the model or trust the client."

"I get that, and I'm aware that might be the job of the Ivana-who-isn't-a-part together with the client's Self."

(Like a therapist during direct access would update a client's part about who the client is now, as a supervisor, I begin to update this therapist part about Self's existence, role, and effect in the therapeutic relationship.) "It might not be your job or within your power to get all those parts to trust you, the model, and the client."

"So, what can I do?"

(I consider I have permission to continue updating the part about Self and Self's capabilities compared to the part's own.) "Well, the more your energy is there in sessions with this client, the more it feeds his 'knowing' part's energy. It's like you feed off each other's energy." (The supervisee is nodding in agreement with this.) "Unfortunately, that isn't as healing. Instead, Ivana's Self could attract or help evoke Paddy's Self who can heal exiles. So, you can help Ivana and Paddy most by giving space."

"Okay, I get that. But I don't think Self is enough."

"Sure, and the help you've given is really valuable. All that knowledge you've gathered and hold." (Appreciating the part's contribution is important and I'm hopeful the supervisee will continue the appreciation using insight once I hand over to the supervisee's Self.) "Would you like to meet the Ivana who isn't a part?"

"Yes."

"Great ... Ivana, do you sense the part?" (Nodding) "How do you feel toward this part?"

"Grateful, I appreciate it holding the knowledge and information, and it can feed that to me from behind." (Ivana is gesticulating as she talks) "I sense the part out beyond the back of my head."

(Wanting to check on the Self-to-part connection, I ask,) "Who does the part see when it looks at you?"

"Light and energy – it's a bit awestruck. I can feel the energy in me."

"Great. Notice that energy and help the part notice and feel that energy ... Ivana, how was it for the part, your suggestion to work together?"

"I heard *Yes* from the part; *we'd make a good team/partnership ...*" (The supervisee is coming back to the room.) "That was magic."

(We are nearing the end of the session, so I ask the supervisee to mentally turn back toward the client.)

"And do you have a sense of how to proceed with the client?"

"If feels much clearer now, no fogginess."

(I ask Ivana to send final appreciation for now to her hardworking therapist part and wait as she opens her eyes.)

By working vertically (up and down the supervisee sidebar of the psychotherapeutic H), we have sought a protector's explicit buy-in to a working alliance with the supervisee's Self. This helps the part have a viable alternative to the part-to-part relationship (represented by the horizontal crossbar of the psychotherapeutic H), in which parts in the supervisee and client had formed an alliance (unconscious, or at least unspoken). Naturally, follow-through work is needed by the supervisee to take this back into their practice, to flesh out the inner working alliance. By following up on how this inner relationship develops and how that development affects the therapeutic relationship, I would also "back up" this supervision session (Williams, 1995, p. 47).

The main purpose of Facet 6 of IFS supervision is to explore and facilitate the multilevel relationship between client and therapist. This may involve uncovering therapist blind spots and biases as well as bringing the unconscious into consciousness.

Facet 7: The Supervisory Relationship

Facet 7 is represented in Figure 14.3 by the diagonal line joining the therapist's system of parts and Self and the supervisor's system of parts and Self. Supervisor and supervisee can focus on and assess the pH or "psychotherapeutic H" of the supervisory relationship (see Figure 14.7). The vertical sidebars of the H refer to the ability of the supervisor and supervisee each to be their own "I" in the storm (Schwartz & Sweezy, 2020) such that each can achieve Self-to-part relationships within their own systems and get to know their own parts. The crossbar of the H draws attention to who in each pair is relating to who in the other at any moment. It reminds us to reflect on the ability of the supervisor and supervisee to relate to the other from Self, speak for not from parts, and have parts relax/step back as required.

Also, as the one (usually) with more power, I hold responsibility to enquire explicitly about, and pay conscious attention to, the relationship with my supervisee and our working alliance. Following up on the impact of supervision may also be considered part of the supervisor's role (Williams, 1995).

The main purpose of this aspect of supervision is to explore and facilitate the potentially multifaceted relationship between therapist and supervisor. This may include noticing and naming how dynamics in the supervisory dyad may mirror dynamics in the therapeutic dyad. For those who feel drawn to exploring this facet, on their website, CSTD London (2021) offers the free resource of a self, peer, supervisor, and supervisee enquiry form.

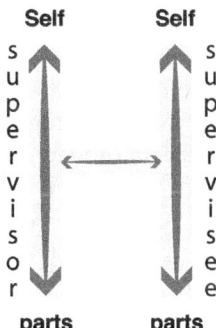

Figure 14.7 The Supervisory Dyad and the Psychotherapeutic H (pH)

Examples of where strain sometimes occurs in my own supervisory relationships include:

- Lack of some aspects of contracting, particularly around expectations, and the likelihood and value of rupture and repair processes.
- Parts in supervisees being exiled or denied and equivalent parts in my system overworking or becoming activated.
- Role conflict, for example when called upon to evaluate therapist competency and performance, which triggers parts who do not want to be "the expert" or "the judge," while other parts take such gatekeeping responsibilities seriously.
- Negotiating changes to the supervisory contract, and when one or both of us has parts triggered by a difference between us.

Self-supervision or supervision of supervision can be useful if supervisor parts are overly active in a supervisory relationship.

Facet 7 supervision questions include:

- What parts are relating or being triggered in the supervisory relationship?
- Where does unblending and/or building internal Self-to-part relationship need to be given attention?
- How do I feel toward the supervisee/supervisor?
- What is not being said between us?
- What conscious and unconscious biases, expectations, and assumptions might we each hold, and what impact are they having in the relationship?

See also *In Love with Supervision* for an inquiry process that focuses on the supervisory relationship (Shohet & Shohet, 2020, ch. 7).

Facet 8: The Wider System(s)

This eighth facet of IFS supervision reminds us to hold in mind the systemic understanding that, at the organizational, community, cultural, national, and even global levels, managers, firefighters, and exiles exist with their polarities, alliances, and cultural and legacy burdens, together with Self. Schwartz and Sweezy (2020, ch. 18) apply the IFS model to social and cultural systems. They write about "the 'person' of the United States" (2020, p. 241) in whom Self-leadership seems obscured by exiles, firefighters, and managers whose experiences have been shaped by legacy burdens of racism, patriarchy, materialism, and individualism. In the film *The Wisdom of Trauma* (Benazzo et al., 2021), Dr. Gabor Maté seems to recognize one of the triadic clusters of parts in Western society as follows: managers: capitalism; firefighters: addicts; exiles: the traumatized.

Focusing on this facet in IFS supervision is likely to include working with issues of diversity and inclusion and implicit bias (see Chapter 9 by Kate Lingren, Chapter 12 by Roberta Rachel Omin, and Chapter 7 by Jeanne Catanzaro), activism, spirituality, and interconnectedness. In Chapter 10, Mary Steege includes a figure template showing interconnected systems onto which a consultee or client can plot parts, Self, specific legacy burdens, etc.

Viewing from this facet might involve attending to and hope merchanting around the interconnectedness of all beings and nature as well as the ubiquity of Self. Merritt (2021, p. 754) writes, "humans do not think of themselves as being part of nature. We are the only species that has to consciously be aware of this basic fact."

The main purpose of this facet of supervision is to take a broader perspective of the systems within which individual systems are nested and to reflect on the impact of context on all systems, processes, and relationships.

Facet 8 supervision questions include:

- What cultural and personal legacy burdens are present in the therapeutic and supervisory systems? What is their impact?
- How is bias experienced/hidden/expressed by parts in the therapeutic and supervisory systems?
- How are issues of power and control showing up or hidden in any of the interconnected systems?
- How is difference (of culture, color, gender, status, and so on) experienced/hidden or ignored/communicated by parts in the therapeutic and supervisory systems?
- What are the expectations of the wider context(s) around the supervision relationship?
- How do I, my supervisees, and their clients experience the interconnectedness (or not) of all things?

Conclusion

In answer to the question I posed at the start of this chapter, I can turn toward fearful (and all) parts in my system and in the other's system from a place of curiosity and permission without an agenda to change or banish them. I am becoming the "I" in my storm, and my pH balance is improving. Two of my supervision trainers write, "Validate the place of anxiety and make it a function of what is happening between supervisor and supervisee" (Shohet & Wilmot, 1991). I am learning it makes sense that anxiety and fear accompany us or arise in us during supervision and that I can be mindful of fear and shame, which may be hidden or going unseen (Mearns, 1991) in any of the participants of supervision.

Session by session, relationship by relationship, I am learning to navigate the 8 Facets and the Fs and Ps (Chapter 3) of IFS supervision. Although attending to any facet may include facilitating a supervisee in doing their own inner work, it is important for me to remind myself, my supervisees, and the readers of this book that, ultimately, supervision is for the benefit of the client – yet not solely for the benefit of the client.

It is my hope that this model and this book will shine a light on IFS supervision and its contributions to there being more Self-energy and Self-leadership in the therapy room and in the world. May fewer parts feel the need to hide and may "the invisibles" in our societies be seen (Merritt, 2021, p. 755). Furthermore, as news reports indicate that global warming has reached the unstoppable tipping point, may humanity and wider global political systems begin to see more clearly our interconnectedness with nature and respond accordingly. In this Anthropocene Era that Merritt (2021) writes of, seeing with new eyes or clearer vision is more likely to happen, and happen with action, if we can look within and beneath the surface to access Self and to see from Self. Robin DiAngelo (2019) writes that a pier seen from an aerial viewpoint looks like it floats on the surface of the water. Rather, it is held up by pillars that cannot be seen from above. Similarly, from one view, we humans appear to be "mono" and "separate." Yet, from an IFS viewpoint, each of us is multiple, and we are each connected to the other, to Larger Self, part of nature, the earth and beyond.

Note

1 Excerpt from *No Bad Parts: Healing Trauma and Restoring Wholeness with the Internal Family Systems Model* © 2021 Richard Schwartz, Ph.D., used with permission from the publisher, Sounds True Inc.

References

Axline, V. M. (1964). *Dibs in search of self: Personality development in play therapy.* Penguin.

Benazzo, Z., Benazzo, M., & Harrison, C. (Directors). (2021). *The wisdom of trauma: Featuring Dr. Gabor Maté* [Film]. Science & Nonduality, & The Hive Studios.

Bolton, R. (1979). *People skills: How to assert yourself, listen to others, and resolve conflicts.* Prentice-Hall.

Brown, B. (2017). *Braving the wilderness: The quest for true belonging and the courage to stand alone.* Vermillion.

CSTD London. (2021, September 27). *Self/peer/supervisor/supervisee enquiry.* https://view.officeapps.live.com/op/view.aspx?src=https%3A%2F%2Fwww.cstdlondon.co.uk%2Fwp-content%2Fuploads%2F2020%2F06%2Fenquiry-form.docx&wdOrigin=BROWSELINK.

Felitti, V. J., Anda, R. F., Nordenberg, D., Williamson, D. F., Spitz, A. M., Edwards, V., Koss, M. P., & Marks, J. S. (1998). Relationship of childhood abuse and household dysfunction to many of the leading causes of death in adults. The Adverse Childhood Experiences (ACE) Study. *American journal of preventive medicine.* 14(4), 245–258. doi:10.1016/s0749-3797(98)00017-8.

DiAngelo, R. (2019). *White fragility: Why it's so hard for white people to talk about racism.* Penguin.

Gilbert, M., & Evans, K. (2000). *Psychotherapy supervision.* Open University Press.

Hawkins, P., & Shohet, R. (2012). *Supervision in the helping professions.* Open University Press.

Hawthorne, L. (1975). Games supervisors play. *Social work, 20*(3),179–183.

Hughes, L. & Pengelly, P. (1997). *Staff supervision in a turbulent environment: Managing process and task in front-line services.* Jessica Kingsley.

Kadushin, A., & Harkness, D. (2014). *Supervision in social work* (5th ed.). Columbia University Press.

Karpman, S. (1968). Fairy tales and script drama analysis. *Transactional Analysis Bulletin, 7*(26), 39–43.

Kinsey Institute Traumatic Stress Research Consortium. (2020). *Kinsey Institute Traumatic Stress Research Consortium Newsletter.* Indiana University. https://kinseyinstitute.org/pdf/TSRC_Newsletter_2_3.20.2020.pdf.

Mearns, D. (1991). On being a supervisor. In W. Dryden & B. Thorne (Eds.), *Training and supervision for counselling in action* (pp. 116–128). Sage.

Merritt, D. (2021). George Floyd's death and COVID-19: Inflection points in the Anthropocene Era? *Journal of Analytical Psychology, 66*(3), 750–762. doi:10.1111/1468-5922.12675.

Proctor, B., & Tehrani, N. (2001). Issues for counsellors and supporters. In N. Tehrani (Ed.), *Building a culture of respect: Managing bullying at work* (pp. 221–224). Taylor and Francis.

Rappoport, A. (2005). Co-narcissism: How we accommodate to narcissistic parents. *Alan Rappoport, PhD, Psychotherapy: Theory and Practice.* http://www.alanrappoport.com/pdf/Co-Narcissism%20Article.pdf.

Redfern, E. E. (2021). The Drama Triangle and Healthy Triangle in supervision. *The Irish Journal of Counselling and Psychotherapy 21*(1): 4–8.

Rennie, D. L. (1994). Clients' deference in psychotherapy. *Journal of Counselling Psychology, 41*(4), 427–437.

Schwartz, R. C. (1995). *Internal Family Systems therapy.* The Guilford Press.

Schwartz, R. C. (2013). The therapist–client relationship and the transformative power of Self. In M. Sweezy & E. L. Ziskind (Eds.), *Internal Family Systems therapy: New dimensions* (pp. 1–23). Routledge.

Schwartz, R. C. (2021). *No bad parts.* Sounds True.

Schwartz, R. C., & Sweezy, M. (2020). *Internal Family Systems therapy* (2nd ed.). The Guilford Press.

Shohet, R., & Shohet, J. (2020). *In love with supervision: Creating transformative conversations.* PCCS Books.

Shohet, R., & Shohet, J. (2021, January). Supervision as spiritual practice. *Thresholds.* BACP.

Shohet, R., & Wilmot, J. (1991). The key issue in the supervision of counsellors: The supervisory relationship. In W. Dryden & B. Thorne, *Training and supervision for counselling in action* (pp. 87–98). Sage.

St. Arnaud, K. O. (2017). Encountering the wounded healer: Parallel process and supervision. *Canadian Journal of Counselling and Psychotherapy, 51*(2), 131–144.

Sykes, C. (2017). An IFS lens on addiction: Compassion for extreme parts. In M. Sweezy & E. L. Ziskind (Eds.), *Innovations and elaborations in Internal Family Systems therapy* (pp. 29–48). Routledge.

Wheeler, S. (2007). What shall we do with the wounded healer? The supervisor's dilemma. *Psychodynamic practice, 13*(3), 245–256.

Williams, A. (1995). *Visual and active supervision: Roles, focus, technique.* Norton.

Glossary

5 Ps	The qualities of someone who is Self-led: Presence, Perspective, Patience, Persistence, and Playfulness. The 5 Ps are especially useful for a therapist to embody in a therapeutic relationship.
6 Fs	Initial healing steps taken to differentiate and get to know a part: (1) Find, (2) Focus, (3) Flesh out, (4) (how do you) Feel toward?, (5) beFriend, and (6) (explore the part's) Fears.
8 Cs	The core qualities of Self: Curiosity, Calm, Compassion, Courage, Confidence, Clarity, Creativity, and Connectedness. They are central to the non-pathologizing, accepting nature of IFS professionals.
Burdens	The sensations, bodily restrictions, or extreme or outdated beliefs about self, the other, and the world carried by parts and arising from times when a person was hurt, terrified, abandoned, neglected, shamed, invalidated, or was met with lack of attunement. They can be **personal burdens**, which arise from the part's own experience, or **legacy burdens**, which have been passed down from a parent or authority figure and arise from the experience of that person or someone of a previous generation. **Cultural burdens** are those that come into a person's system from their culture. All burdens lead to imbalance and cause constraints in systems.
Categories of parts	*Part* is the term IFS uses for the subpersonalities inside of us, and each part has its own thoughts, feelings, behaviors, memories, and experiences. There are two main categories of part: protectors and exiles. IFS subdivides protectors into **managers** and **firefighters**, while **exiles** tend to be those they protect. Parts may be very young, and all can carry burdens.
Differentiation	An important concept in IFS that refers to the processes of distinguishing different parts from each other and from Self, distinguishing a part from its burden or role, or distinguishing one kind of burden from another, as well as the past from the present and the future.

DOI: 10.4324/9781003044864-15

Direct Access	The alternative approach to in-sight. When a protector will not unblend or an exile is overwhelming the system, the therapist speaks directly to the unblended part. *Explicit* direct access is when we speak to a part and make it explicit that this is what we are doing (e.g., "Can I talk to that part directly? Hello, how are you trying to help Nathan when he's with his client?"). *Implicit* direct access is used when the person is fully blended with a part, rejects the idea of parts, or says, "What do you mean, 'step back,' this is me?" Then we speak to the part without overtly acknowledging that this what we are doing.
Exiles	Parts, usually young and trapped in the past, that the protectors are dedicated to keeping out of everyday life and consciousness. Exiles carry the pain, memories, and beliefs of past hurts. When unburdened, they can return to their naturally healthy states.
Firefighters	Parts functioning as the secondary, reactive line of defense that take charge when managerial strategies fail. Firefighters can use extreme behaviors and, for this reason, are often not well-liked by the managers, who may fear the consequences of such extreme behaviors. Firefighter strategies include soothing and distracting.
Healing Steps	Healing Steps include: (1) the **6 Fs**, (2) **Witnessing**, (3) **Redo (or Do-Over)**, (4) **Retrieval**, (5) **Unburdening**, (6) **Invitation**, and (7) **Integration (and Appreciation)**.
Hope merchant(ing)	Part of the role and one of the skills of the IFS professional is to actively hold the possibility of inner healing and transformation of parts (if they allow it) and then offer ("sell") that hope in a Self-led way to client's parts such that they can open themselves to new possibilities.
In-sight	The primary approach used in IFS with adults to get to know and understand parts. In-sight requires that the person be aware of parts and have enough Self-energy to communicate with them directly, either in the internal world or externally if the part is represented externally. When protectors won't separate or an exile is hijacking the person's system and unblending is not possible, direct access may be needed.
Integration (and Appreciation)	The final healing step in which the person's Self invites protectors to notice how the exile has changed (unburdened, healed, and in potentially closer connection with Self and the rest of the system). Self offers appreciation for what the protector has done for the system, including giving space for the exile's healing, and helps the protector let go of any burdens they carry, find a new role in the system, and/or take a rest.

Invitation   A healing step in which an unburdened part invites in qualities it wants or needs for the future to take the place of the burden (s) it let go. One or more of the **8 Cs** of Self are commonly chosen.

Larger Self (sometimes SELF)   The term used to signify the less individual, more expansive and inclusive or transcendent nature of Self. It can be thought of as the source from which Self and Self-energy come in the way that the *Imago Dei* (image of God) or Buddha Nature are terms for that aspect of the supreme principle or ground of being in the universe contained within humanity.

Managers   Parts acting as the primary line of proactive defense, whose job is to stay focused on maintaining normal functioning, stability, and performance (or at least the appearance of these things). This frequently involves exiling emotions and vulnerability and may include the use of various well-intended tactics, such as shaming, criticizing, living in the head, and exiling the body.

Part   *Part* is the term IFS uses for the subpersonalities inside of us, and each part has its own thoughts, feelings, behaviors, memories, and experiences (See Categories of Parts, Managers, Firefighters, and Exiles).

Polarization   The term given to parts (or groups of parts) in conflict often showing up as protectors competing over how to protect or avoid an exile. A polarization may become more extreme as each side fears their opponent(s) taking control. Polarizations take up a lot of energy in a system, block access to Self, and distract from approaching and healing exiles. Inner polarities impact external systems and can evoke parts in others, who polarize (or form an alliance) across systems with the other's parts. It is beneficial to facilitate Self's relationship with polarized parts, including acknowledging the contributions and intentions of each part (or group) and negotiating for Self-leadership. This can increase inner harmony by helping protectors relax and paves the way for healing of exiles.

Redo (or Do-Over)   A healing step in which, in order to leave the past, the exiled part may want or need something different to happen back then, and it can have the Self (usually of the person but also potentially of the therapist) enter the scene to do or say or have done what it needed at the time. In addition, the presence of Self may enable the part itself to complete anything it was unresourced or unable to complete or do differently at the time.

Retrieval   A healing step where the Self of the person helps the exiled part out of the scene in which it is stuck and brings it to the present or a fantasy place where it wants to be.

Self The term used to describe the innate presence in each of us
(Self-energy) that is the only inner entity fully resourced to lead the internal family and bring transformation and healing. Self cannot be damaged or destroyed and continues to exist when parts constrain Self by blending and taking over the seat of consciousness. In IFS the qualities of Self are highlighted by the **8 Cs** and the **5 Ps**. Self-energy is sometimes experienced as spaciousness, tingling, warmth, light, and energy. Together with C and P qualities, extending Self-energy to parts helps build a relationship between Self and part(s).

Self- When a person's system is led by a Self who hears, validates,
leadership and is in relationship with parts, acknowledging and appreciating each part's role and contribution, internally and in the world. Self-leadership fluctuates.

Trailhead The point at which a path or trail begins. In IFS, a trailhead is the initial awareness offering us a path inside (perhaps through noticing a thought, emotion, body sensation, extreme reaction, memory, impulse, or urge) that leads to a part.

Unburdening The healing step that is the summation of the transformation process: in its basic form the exiled part takes the burden from in, on, or around its body and chooses how to release it—typically to one of the elements air, earth, fire, light, or water or in a ceremony of its choice.

U-Turn The process/act of turning one's attention away from the other person or persons and the external world and directing curiosity toward one's own internal world and reactivity.

Witnessing A healing step in which the Self of the person witnesses and really "gets" whatever the part wants to share about its experience from its own perspective (this may or may not be shared with a third party, such as the therapist or consultant). Feeling understood, accepted, and loved by Self in this way can be a moving and powerfully transformative experience.

Appendix: Methods for Unblending

Dan Reed and Ray Wooten

Being Curious or U-Turning

U-turning is making our reactivity our business. Rather than blaming and putting energy into making the outside situation or person change, we invite curiosity inside the person who is uncomfortable/struggling and begin to wonder and develop a relationship with that discomfort inside that person. This way of becoming curious is invaluable in being with ourselves as consultants and supervisors, inviting therapists or anyone else we are working with to wonder about their own reactivity.

Examples of U-turn type questions (Herbine-Blank et al., 2015; Reed, 2019):

> What's happening inside or around your body?
> What is it afraid/concerned would happen if it didn't do this?
> Who is that part looking at (or focusing on)?
> How are you feeling toward your client/this part of your client?
> Who does that part think that you are?
> What is that part of you saying about you, the other person, and/or your relationship?
> What would it do for you if the other person would … ?

> - How would that help you?
> - What would the hope be if they would do that?
> - Who would that help?

Pausing

This is often the first step in a U-turn. Either the consultant or therapist can request a pause to slow down and become curious about themselves or the process they find themselves in.

Blending to Unblend (Direct Access)

The consultant implicitly allows or explicitly invites a part to (mostly or fully) blend with the therapist. (In its more extreme forms, blending is also known as "hijacking" or "overwhelming" when it happens without invitation.) This invitation can help facilitate that part feeling seen, heard, and sensed from its perspective by the therapist's Self and the Self of the consultant or supervisor. As the part feels more known, it is then more likely to unblend and give more space for the therapist's Self.

Note: Direct Access Fluidly Flows into In-Sight

With direct access, the consultant engages directly with a part that is mostly or fully blended with the therapist to support the part in feeling seen, heard, and sensed from its perspective(s). As the part is experienced from its perspective, more space opens up, differentiating the therapist's Self from their part(s). The therapist naturally becomes less blended and more Self-led, and in-sight becomes a fluid next step in further developing Self–part reciprocal relationship. In-sight is a process of the therapist's Self relating directly with their own parts and speaking for and advocating for their parts' experiences.

Externalizing: An Alternate Form of In-Sight

With externalizing, the consultant encourages the therapist to use something outside of their body to represent their part(s) in order to unblend from those parts and develop direct relationship with them. Externalizing is actually the same process as in-sight, only the therapist can physically see the part represented outside of them and sense the three-dimensional physical/spatial relationship between them. Examples of methods to externalize include sculpting (using real people to represent parts), using a sandtray or small world objects, parts mapping, placing objects around the therapist that represent the parts, or dialoguing with an empty chair.

Consultant Teaching Skills to Therapists

Teaching can be a useful way for consultants to unblend from their own parts when they are either knowingly or unknowingly activated. Teaching allows some of the consultant's manager parts to feel some more confidence, competence, and clarity, while slowing the process down and creating space for the consultant's system to settle.

Teaching and skills practice can also be a fantastic way to slow down the process and allow parts of a therapist to start to trust that there is a plan and they don't needs to be so scared. Perhaps the therapist actually lacks the skills and needs practice/information for their parts to relax, or perhaps a cluster of scared parts needs the consultant to guide the therapist through something to see and confirm that the therapist already knows how to do this, and then the therapist's parts can relax.

Inviting Playfulness

The consultant being playful can deflate some of the heavy seriousness and trapped feelings that therapist parts can experience when those parts feel scared, pressured, or burdened by responsibility. Humor, levity, and poking fun at the gravitas that isn't the therapist's or consultant's to carry can shake things up just enough for the therapist's parts to soften and for the therapist to gain a larger perspective.

Reflecting Using Parts Language

> "I'm hearing that part of you … "
> "Sounds like something in you … "
> "Can you sense the sadness in there?"

Whether saying "part of" or using more everyday language, the consultant using parts language points toward something within a therapist's experience. This step in supporting a therapist to differentiate from their parts can make the therapist's experience of their challenges feel proportionately smaller and creates space for the possibility of relating with the experience/feeling/part in the present moment.

Speaking for Parts

> "Part of me … "
> "I can sense some [insert feeling word], it's … "
> "I have mixed feelings … "

Saying "A part of me …" or describing an internal experience both acknowledges and advocates for parts and creates a possibility for parts to know they are not alone. Something other than them (Self) is looking out for them.

Asking for Parts That Are Blending to Make Space and Wait

> "Ask that part to step back."
> "Ask this one that's coming in right now if it would be willing to watch for a little while."
> "Maybe the one who's trying to figure all this out could hang back and watch for a little so we can help it get some new information. How does that sound to it?"

This direct communication with parts lets them know that someone else is here, that someone is aware of them, and that someone else is willing and wanting to lead.

Developing Ongoing Relationships (Before, During, and After Sessions)

Therapists learning the "tells" (somatic markers, voice tone, thought patterns, feelings, preferences, etc.) of when particular parts are present can be invaluable for getting in relationship with a particular part in the present moment. Also checking in before and after session for parts' concerns or how things went from their perspective can help strengthen trust and develop relationships with parts that tend to get activated in or by the therapist's sessions.

References

Herbine-Blank, T., Kerpelman, D., & Sweezy, M. (2015). *Intimacy from the Inside Out*. Routledge.

Reed, D. A. (2019). Internal Family Systems informed supervision: A grounded theory inquiry (Identifier ETD2019Reed). Doctoral Dissertation, *St. Mary's University Digital Commons Repository*. https://commons.stmarytx.edu/dissertations/27.

Index

Page numbers in **bold** refer to tables, and page numbers in *italics* refer to figures
In this index, the terms "consultant" "consultee" and "consultation," are used as "umbrella" terms. If an entry points to text about American-style supervision or material written by a UK author, "supervision" terms are used.

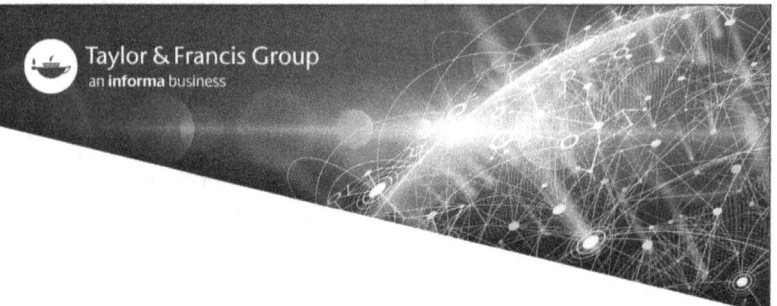
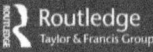
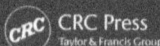